I CRY FOR HELP!

I CRY FOR HELP!

◆

Autobiography/Health, My True Story Detailing the Aftermath of Child Abuse, Trauma, Stress, Combat Trauma, & Post Traumatic Stress Disorder

PHIL DORMAN

iUniverse, Inc.
New York Lincoln Shanghai

I CRY FOR HELP!

Autobiography/Health, My True Story Detailing the Aftermath of Child Abuse, Trauma, Stress, Combat Trauma, & Post Traumatic Stress Disorder

iUniverse books may be ordered through booksellers or by contacting:

iUniverse
2021 Pine Lake Road, Suite 100
Lincoln, NE 68512
www.iuniverse.com
1-800-Authors (1-800-288-4677)

The information, ideas and suggestions in this book are not intended as a substitute for professional medical advice. Before following any suggestions contained in this book, you should first consult your personal physician.
Neither the author nor the publisher shall be liable or responsible for any loss or damage allegedly arising as a consequence of your use or application of any information or suggestions in this book.

ISBN-13: 978-0-595-40961-7 (pbk)
ISBN-13: 978-0-595-85320-5 (ebk)
ISBN-10: 0-595-40961-X (pbk)
ISBN-10: 0-595-85320-X (ebk)

Printed in the United States of America

Contents

CHAPTER 4   What Are Intrusive Narratives (In) or

CHAPTER 5   Are They Physical Or Mental Ailments?.......... 65

Prologue

My name is Phil Dorman. The disorders that malign me are acute Post Traumatic Stress Disorder (PTSD) with many symptoms of Dissociative Disorders (DD) and Bi-polar. My dear wife and I being wed for thirty-two years shows our commitment to each other. For more than ten years, we have suffered the affects of these plagues and disorders. Everyone in our family has endured much more, than I would have liked. Every close nit groups eventually incurs legal or medical problems and that's only two events that have completely devastated our family unit. During the pressures of these circumstances, family members should provide support. We didn't receive any type of family support.

I'm not a doctor or in the medical profession. So, don't look for any twenty-five cent words. This style of writing doesn't place another layer of confusion to an already complex issue. Everyone may relax for this book is exam free.

We have spent many days and night praying for the answers about PTSD. Exactly like your family, we are trying to understand what we will face with PTSD. We don't have the rest of our lives to wait for the correct answers to fall out of the sky. I thought here is the good place for saying the knowledge I've received is not like on the job training. I want to share the wealth of knowledge and understanding we've found with you and your loved ones. This knowledge has given me the strength to begin coping with the challenges presented by PTSD. Learning coping skills was an important key for both my family and me. I say that, because the person with PTSD may not always be able to understand or cope. Personally, I have endured ten years of random episodes and each one has been different. The PTSD episodes are unpredicted. The person undergoing this extremely rapid mental transformation; requires understanding and assurances, which only love ones and caregivers can provide. This person is full of apprehension, fear, and an array of mood changes in their mental state. First, the person needs enough time to absorb what has happened. This is not easy, most of the time they have no idea of which side of the tracks they're on or even if they are in a hallucination or reality. As the caregiver can bring calm and peace, for the may be delirious, displaced, overcome by fear, and worrying about finances. All of this could be like me, my mind was racing or speeding at such a rate that the processing part of my brain could not keep pace.

Becoming ill these were some of the questions, I needed immediate answers. What was the cause of my illness? What is happening to me? How do I stop? Am I going to die from this? How long will it be until I am well enough to go back to work? Well, I cannot tell you there is any quick fix. This is a very complex disease, to state it mildly. Not being able to predict what or when something will occur causes an extreme anxiety that overcomes the mind.

This disease is incurable, but not hopeless. The use of coping skills is the best we can hope for presently. The severity of PTSD is the key to each person's recovery. As with the severity, there are also different levels of recovery. These things I have learned from years of therapy. You can do some immediate things. Calm down and learn to understand the disease you're working with. In that way you are not, surprised by each change you observe. This book will provide some of the answers, for which you're searching. Finally, this book has been written that helps you understand through true life experiences. This is not a technical book in anyway! I think a person who has PTSD can explain exactly what this disease does inside the body and mind best.

I found that when I first became ill, I was scared to death! I've been in war conditions and PTSD conditions were more terrifying to me. In war conditions, I knew what the rules and game plan was. With PTSD, I had no such knowledge to obtain the rules. Everybody knows that you can't play the game, if you don't know the rules. I could not understand what was going on around me.

The challenges for me were to understand speech and explain the things I heard that no one else heard. Systematically, I lost control of my speech, hearing, and sight. Drink and eating was almost impossible. Erratically, I lost control of my legs, arms, or body. From my point of view, no one could communicate with me nor I with them. There was no way for me to talk to anyone. Without success, I tried to write on paper, so my family would know what was happening. They couldn't read what I wrote. My ability to spell was gone. My temper was at the point of explosion. What was I to do? What was going on? Whom could I trust? Even I couldn't understand what was going on inside my own mind. There were very big questions and very few answers. Everything felt so strange to me and I was very paranoid. There was a battle in my mind, I did not know if I could trust my own wife. Somehow, I was under the notion that she was going to poison me. I thought that if I went to sleep or got in the shower, the men in the white coats were going to come and take me away. Keep in mind all of these changes occurred overnight! PTSD is not a disease like a cold or the flu, which slowly gets worse, until you're very sick.

In this book, I hope by sharing my real life illustrations of the PTSD symptoms. The people with PTSD and their families can learn to cope with many everyday situations. Believe me I don't have all the answers, but I think I can share quite a few. In order to protect the dignity and privacy of other names have been changed.

Written: January 16, 2002 by Phil Dorman

1

This Is What Happened To Me!

A True Story

I am going to show you the words written in my journal the day I became ill. No one in my family had any idea something was wrong. No one saw it coming. This is what happened to me! It all seems to have come from a thriller movie script. It wasn't until later that the star of the movie was exposed.

It was May 7, 1995. A sunny day as I remember. As always sitting at my computer, the place my family could always find me. Peering out the window in my office it was nice to watch my huskies play. A very strong headache captured my attention. This was the worst headache in resent memory. Sitting in a captain's chair my body began getting numb. While thinking my feet and legs were going to sleep, wondering what the matter was I tried to turn them from side to side. Then, without warning, my entire body became numb. Fear started to grip me, as something appeared on the office wall. With eyes squinted, I saw a distinct image on the wall. This cannot be I closed by eyes, and the image remained the same. I didn't know what it was. It looked like some kind of drawing or image. Never had I seen anything like this in my life. OK now, taking a deep breath saying logic must prevail. It's on the wall, when I look there. It's in front of my eyes, when I close them. Yes, I'm really freaking out now! For safety sake, I disconnected from the multiple computer systems I had logged on to and shut down my own computer. My loving wife came in sometime later and asked kindly, "What was wrong?" Just sitting in my chair gazing at this image on the wall was not a normal activity to engage my thoughts.

I pointedly asked her, do…"Do you see something on the wall?" We talked a bit and I told her about my headache, how I was feeling, and the image on the wall. She asked, "What image on the wall is it you're watching?" That response made me think I was loosing it completely!

The same sequence of events happened on the following day. My headache was so bad; that lying down on the bed seem the only solution. This must be a

1

migraine headache. Going to the doctor seemed like the next logical step if this continues! Never had I been so impressed to seek the assistance of a doctor. Most of the time home remedies worked just fine for me. I saw the same strange image on multiple occasions. The second viewing and immediately recognition of the image, remove any sense of fear. My concern grew, but I didn't want to alarm my wife. I thought that later 'I'd check it out' and everything would be all right. As normal, I went to work on May 9, 1995.

Well, the 'old check it out later', was not such a good idea. On May 10, 1995, this date will stick in my mind forever, something even stranger happened to me!

On this date, my responsibilities centered as a Computer Scientist. Auxiliary duties included support as a Systems Administrator. My responsibility was to take care of over one hundred fifty computers connected to a high-speed fiber network. The 4 PM to 12 AM shift was my regular hours for work.

On Wednesday, I awoke at my normal time. I made coffee; my wife had already gone to work. It felt like it was just a normal workday. I was feeling all right. Then, all of a sudden, a very strange feeling came over me. A chill began to flow over my entire body. Immediately, I began taking notes about what was happening to me!

The Following Is An Exact Copy Of The Writing Before I Froze Up On May 10, 1995. Please Excuse The Spelling And Logic Within The Sentences:

"5/10 Wed—woke up at 9 am—now 10:30 am. Felt confused…took pill for headache. My mind is still asleep, but my body is awake. This feeling started over the weekend. This feeling went away by Sunday night. Now…feel…lost, alone, no direction, confused, and afraid.…This happened on the weekend also. Then a loud crack sound went off in my head, felt sick, and then all things were normal again.…. Right now, I feel numb and can't spell or understand what is going on. I feel lost and worried. I wish my mind would wake up; my hands are shaking, feel as though I am on autopilot, doing things, but for no reason—just doing. I thought write this down, so I would remember this to talk to a doctor about what is happening…I feel this is very sad, but can't make it stop. I feel like it is time to go somewhere…getting faint…calling my wife now.… Wife is coming…heart is beating very fast and hard…Help…call work for something or me…no call.… Work…"

I was loosing control and feeling of my body. As the shaking began, I starred at the image with new additions to the three balls linked together by three blue laser lights. Sequentially the loss of control moved from one part of my anatomy to another. First, my legs, the ability to walk, writing, and spelling went out the window. Words now appeared on the paper with large and small letters, and the writing lines were not used. I was getting very scared now! I called my wife at work and when she answered the phone the only word I could say was, "Help." The people at her office again called "911."

When my daughter walked in the house, she saw me stuck in one position in the kitchen chair and I could not talk to her. She asked, "Dad, Dad is something wrong? Is something wrong?" Slowly I nodded my head, "Yes." She asked if she should call "911." Again, I nodded my head, "Yes." My daughter immediately calls 911!

I did not know what was wrong. An ambulance arrived for each "911" call. The medics asked, "What' wrong? What's the problem?" I was answering their questions, but they heard nothing. They wrote down patient not responsive. That's when I realized they could not hear me speak, even though I knew I was speaking.

That's when I notice I still saw the image. (The image is may be found at the end of this section). Looking at the image on the white kitchen cabinet bought out the colors in it. I saw inside the body part, there was a cluster of six red balls, sending red laser beams to the center (seventh) red ball, each time I spoke. The other thing I noted was that the blue laser beams between Mind, Body, and Spirit were not present. Only the three balls were there.

One of the ambulances took my daughter and me to the hospital. When I got there, we had to answer many questions. I thought I was speaking. Again, they wrote patient not responding. The doctor's thought since I could not speak, then I must not be able to hear either. They were completely wrong! They spoke very candidly, right in front of me. I knew what they were planning every step of the way. They did not know what was wrong with me. They thought I must be on some kind of drug. All the tests showed that no drugs were found in my system. They thought aloud, we have to get him signed into the Psychiatric ward. This way they are not liable, if something unfortunate happened to me. They tried to get both my wife and I to sign me into the hospital. The doctors told me that my wife had already signed me in. That's when I felt my wife had betrayed me! I told them that there was no way I was staying in the hospital! I wasn't staying! The doctors had lied to both my wife and I! Somehow, I got enough strength to get myself together, put my cloths on, and get out of there. I could hear them in the background shouting as my wife and I left the hospital, "You'll have to take full responsibility for him, if you take him from this hospital!" My wife, of almost thirty-two years, is my GUARDIAN ANGEL.

When I arrived home, I distrusted everyone. The doctors had totally messed up my thinking. I thought the glue, used to put down the rug, was some kind of poison. I thought the people at work, had put some kind of drug or poison in the pizza we ordered the day before. I went outside of the house on the patio. I just sat there and scared. I didn't know what to do! I could not feel my body. I could not talk. I could not understand what people were saying. I was totally messed up. I did not have any idea about what I should do. Some relatives came, but they did more harm than good. Maybe it was well meaning, but they had no knowledge about what had happened to me. All I can remember is I needed someone I could trust.

"Who could I trust? The one thing to remember is that the person that goes through this (onset of PTSD) they cannot be held accountable for the things the do or say."

I was not capable of making good or bad decisions. My mind was disconnected from my body. This maybe hard to understand, but for me it was truly a nightmare.

On May 11, 1995, my family took me to see a Neurologist. He performed some tests and said he could not help me. He suggested that I go to see a Psychiatrist. During our stay in his office, I became frozen like a statue sitting in a chair.

The only way I have of explaining this to someone is the following: I felt like my body was disconnected from my mind. When this disconnection takes place, my body was frozen in place. I was aware of my surrounds, except I had no ability to interact with anything outside of my mind. This frozen state continues, until my mind can again communicate with my body. It's feels like I'm lockup as a prisoner inside of my own mind.

This happened a few times throughout my wife's conversation with me. My wife told me, that while I was frozen in the chair, the Neurologist did a few tests. The doctor threw a small box at me and I didn't move a muscle. She said I just sat in the chair. The doctor began yelling my name repeatedly. Then, I snapped out of it and returned to the present time.

When I Awoke, It Was As If I Had Gone On A Journey, Somewhere Within My Mind. I didn't know anything about the doctor throwing a box, but I could hear the voices in the room. In addition, it was noted that I could only understand very short sentences. A sentence about three words long. I still could not speak.

On May 12, 1995, I was taken to a medical center to have an MRI performed. I went in the room where a huge MRI machine was waiting. I was placed on a table where I had a complete view of the room. I saw the doctors in a glass booth just a short distance from the end of the table. They talked to me the whole time by microphone from the glass enclosure. They ask if I were ok and they explained the whole procedure. When they were confident, that I understood, they moved the table into the huge cylinder. They tested their microphone and speakers once again. I was assured that they could hear me from with the cylinder. They said to me that they were going to start the process. I told them I was ok. They told me I would hear a slight tapping. I said ok.

Then, All Hell Broke Loose! The whole experience truly took me back in time. I was extremely disoriented, by the loud banging sound made by the machine.

I felt and saw myself back in Vietnam combat engaged in an actual firefight. I was re-experiencing the events from combat, which occurred many years before. It was night and in the dense dark jungle, red tracer bullets coming from everywhere! What I was experiencing, was not just a flashback, this was a full-length continuous running, big screen move, with real action, sight, and sound. The event was completely real to me.

Inside the MRI machine, I told them I had to get out now! I was screaming to them to stop this machine; I have to get out now! (Learning only in the year 2001, this was an experienced was called an intrusive memory). Three attendances came running to secure me to the table. Once the table moved out of the MRI machine, the attendances tried their best to control my movements without success! Uncontrollable, my only desire was to exit the machine and the building! They were explaining that only half of the test was complete. They tried with no success, to explain the second half of the test was to inject some colored die into my veins. Right! I exploded with rage! No one was going to stick anything, anywhere as far as I was concerned. I physically fought like crazy, until I was free! I ran out of the office, like a mad man! My family came out moments later, finding me in front of the medical center holding on with both arms to a column of the building. I was totally out of control! Every bone in my body was shaking as I held on to the column. I was still disoriented not sure, if I was in the present or in the past. It was impossible for me to understand the words my family was speaking! They might as well have been speaking a foreign language. They managed somehow, to get me in the car and take me home.

On May 16, 1995, I saw Dr. Wadeson for the first time. He said he could help me! He gave me some medications and a list of steps, which were written down in bullet form, which I could read to improve my condition. Immediately he gained my trust.

Starting around May 16, 1995, I was not in my right mind for more than six months. Most of my family issues rose from my condition or were related to my lack of ability to comprehend. I was in a different world than everybody else. I was confused, disoriented, felt very low, stupid, depressed, could not read normal sentences, write, work, watch TV, listen to the radio, and almost any form of coherent conversation was impossible for me to participate in or understand.

This is the description of the mind image, as it appeared to me on a few different occasions: Again, from my journal entries dated September 23, 1995:

I saw the image and it was working. When I was thinking about something, lightning would flash in the top ball. A message that looked like a sparkler would travel along the blue laser light to the other two balls. That is why I think the top ball is the mind-thinking center. When I wanted to move a hand or finger a white cell, in the ball labeled body, would light up red and a message that looks like a sparkler would be sent to the other two balls. I believe the third ball must be the spirit, because it contained a vessel.

Created two; three-dimensional models of this image I delivered them to Dr. Wadeson. He sent one copy to the National Institute of Health (NIH) in Washington, D. C. The other copy he kept at his office. The report he received from NIH said, that there were two reports of people seeing a similar image.

The following is a description of each part of the image as written in my journal entries near date of September 23, 1995:

Blue Light (laser): This only appears on the image when things are functioning normally. When they are missing, the patient is sitting staring out into space appearing as stuck or in a trance.

Sparklers: These sparklers travel from the balls labeled Mind, Body, and Spirit carrying messages. The sparklers are always sent when something occurs in any of the balls (Mind, Body, or Spirit). The message sparklers appear like the type of handheld sparkler used on July 4.

Mind: Represented by a flexible ball, which contains a thunderstorm in a cloud. The lightning appears to strike when a person thinks.

Body: Represented by a flexible ball, which contains smaller white balls or cells. There are two types. Independent white balls or cells flash red when activity occurs. There is also, a cluster of six small balls, which turn red when they communicate directly by a red laser light, and into the center or seventh ball or cell. End of journal entry.

Anyone with information about the subject of the image of the mind is cordially invited to share in the investigation. So far, two others have responded having seen similar images.

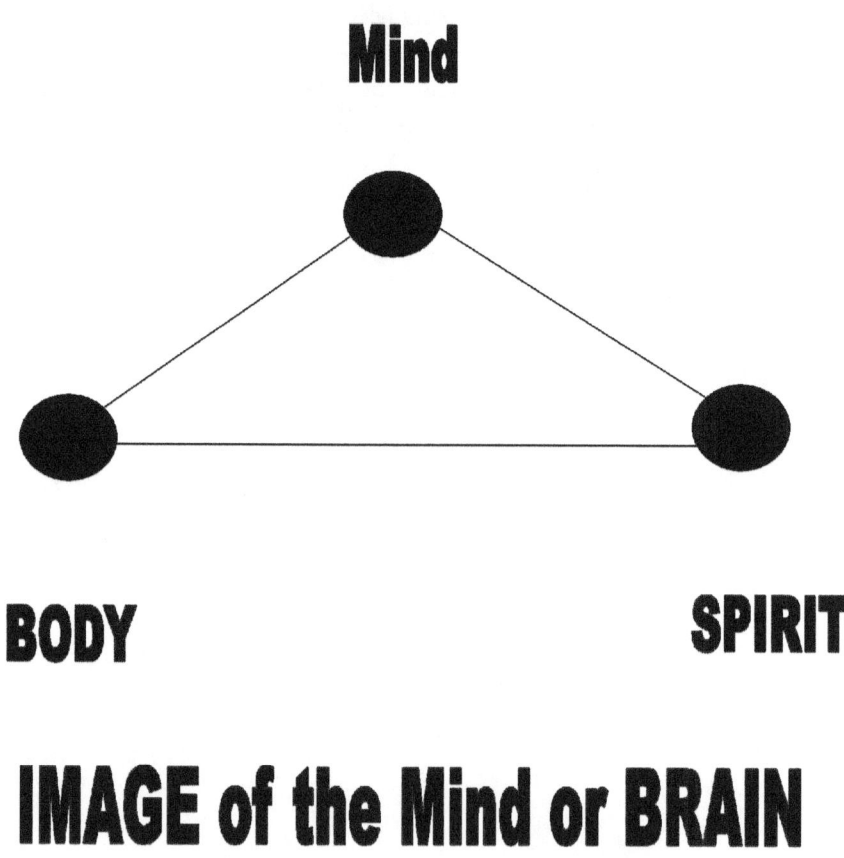

IMAGE of the Mind or BRAIN

Feb. 23, 2002, writing these first few pages has taken me from Dec. 2001 to Feb. 22, 2002. I have had to stop writing many times, because I became very ill and overwhelmed. I didn't want you to think that for me this was an easy task. I have had to push myself through many physical and physiological experiences. To state this in a simple way, I am having a very rough emotional experience writing this book.

The dates next to the section headings show when I was able to finished writing the piece. Dr. Wadeson thought it would be good to show the amount of physical and mental effort it required for me to unscramble all of the thoughts that I'm mentally processing simultaneously. Part of what is being shown is that a person with acute PTSD, can at times, be immobilized by what is occurring inside the brain. Many times, I could not write with a pen, so I typed on the keyboard using one finger.

PROBLEMS CAUSED BY LACK OF KNOWLEDGE—MAR. 24, 2002

Understand that when a person initially has a nervous system shutdown, they are in a very frail mental state. Anyone can easily influence them about any subject. The person is somewhere between reality and unreality. The person doesn't know what is exactly the right or wrong decision to make. They don't have the ability to make an educated discernment of the facts presented. They must rely on those around them, for proper direction and assistance with all decision-making processes. To say it simply, the person is out of it, completely out in the ozone. They cannot be held accountable for the things they do or say. It might be said that they are very gullible and naïve. Let me explain with some of my true-life experiences.

My daughter graduated from high school a few days after I had a nervous system shutdown. My wife and I had agreed months before that, we would present a truck to our daughter as a graduation present. We decided that our daughter had worked very hard for twelve years and accomplished a formidable task.

My family members influenced me by saying that, the truck was too extravagant a gift to give to our daughter. They also told this to my wife and daughter. The news completely devastated my daughter. Every time she looked at the truck, she had only painful reminders of what my relatives told her. All the joy and happiness my wife and I wished for her by giving the truck, was gone. In just a few weeks, she traded the truck in on another vehicle. She couldn't live with the stress caused by having the truck.

My relatives put ideas in my mind, which deeply added to my confusion and made larger problems for my family. They told me that, my daughter and wife were using me for my money. They told me that, my wife was not preparing adequate meals for me. They actually convinced me that, I would be better off under their care and they took me to their house. This was done against the will of my wife, daughter, and Dr. Wadeson. My wife was frantic!

My daughter and wife tried for two week to contact me, but my relative told them they could not speak to me on the phone. My relative told my wife they understood me better. My relative drinks and uses drugs daily. He would say that all I needed was to get a good drink and smoke a little to get a buzz on and that would solve all my problems. I had appointments three times a week with Dr. Wadeson. I had no counseling or medical assistance during the time I was with my relatives. Dr. Wadeson placed me on a number of medications, which had to be monitored closely. There was no monitoring for two weeks. While at my relative's house, they convinced me, that I was sick because my wife was poisoning me. They convinced me that my wife, daughter, and her boyfriend were all threats to me. My relatives insulted my daughter and boyfriend so bad, that my daughter moved out of the house. Her boyfriend is now her husband. One of my relatives was actually pulling my family apart. I guess he succeeded when my daughter left home. I didn't want her or her boyfriend to leave. They were our strongest supporters. "How could this all happen to me?" The whole time all of these things were going on, I thought it was I causing all of the problems and conflicts, but that was a delusion.

My wife had to get Dr. Wadeson to call my whole family into a session to get this mess straightened out. Dr. Wadeson reprimanded my relatives for their actions in the strongest terms. We still don't have contact with any of many relatives to this day. These experiences also, completely overwhelmed by the time I returned home.

The worst part of this for me to bear was that I couldn't remember any of these events happening. This is why I can say, that the person that has a nervous system shutdown will be overwhelmed and completely confused for some period. My confusion has varied from complete to minimum over the past nine years. A health care professional can only determine the level of mental confusion. The above events are a few examples of what "should not" be done! Before doing anything, contact a health care professional and obtain the knowledge needed to address the circumstances. It is possible to make a bad situation worse!

2

My Experiences

DREAM EXPERIENCES

Throughout the last nine years, I have continually been pledged with reoccurring vivid nightmares and dreams. I don't know how to stop them from occurring. My coping tool is to be aware that these dreams happen to everyone and I am not going crazy! This is a very common symptom of PTSD. With my journal next to bed upon awaking, I always wrote down my dreams. Dr. Wadeson has been able to help me interpret some of the dreams. After I have an interpretation of the dream, it seems to go away. This is just another way your brain has of talking to you. Knowing these things would remove some of the fears caused by very vivid strange dreams. I can tell you from my experience; this is not all in your head! Having explained that, these are a few examples of my dreams and journeys.

The Dark Tunnel—Dec. 28, 2002

Lying in my bed asleep, I get an eerie feeling! My body becomes ridged; each joint in my body begins to shake. The jittering continues until my feet, legs, torso, shoulders, arms, and hands are all moving up and down a half an inch or so. A cold chill flows over my body like a bucket of water poured over me. I have a constant pain in the back of my head like a vice crushing my brain. The pain goes down my neck and into my shoulders. The muscles in the back of my neck are so tight I can hear a loud grinding in the center of my head as I turn my head from side to side. There is a great darkness around me. As I look forward, into a deep dark tunnel. The site dumbfounds me. Frozen in my tracks, a sense of being here before surprises me, I was not afraid. The walls seem to narrow as I go farther down the tunnel. Feeling as though I am searching for something specific, a jolt, like something has attached to my back. I am pulled backwards with enormous speed to the entrance of the tunnel. Whisked backward, there is the sound

11

of a strong wind. I am becoming very cold! A loud pop is heard in my ears it pushes my head forward. I awake from sleep, just with my eyes open. Not moving my head, I look from left to right to see where I am. Not knowing where I am, I feel confused, I realize that I am back in my own bedroom lying on my back in bed. I struggle shaking like a leaf to get a cigarette. My dog Jessy is awakened by my jumping and gently lays her head on my leg as if to say, everything will be all right. We both get up to have coffee, while my wife continues to sleep. My wife is used to all this commotion. Many times, she is unaware that anything has happened.

Dream of the Demon Chase—Feb. 4, 2002

Many reoccurring dreams also plague my nights. I will explain exactly what I see when my eyes are closed. Demons chase me for hours at a time. I run across an endless array of pipes. I'm slipping and sliding on mold and condensed water, which is on the surface of the pipes. The walls of this place are made of concrete. The pipes are of all different sizes and they run in all directions as far as I can see. I've never seen any doors or windows to make an escape. The atmosphere is cool and damp. The structure is like a huge, tall tunnel rising up hundreds of feet above me. These demons start chasing me at the bottom of the shaft. Running like a crazy man, I climb from pipe to pipe. There seems to be about four or five demons chasing me. The fiends appear to me as ghastly dark green black blobs. I can see arms and legs as they move about. The evil spirits make a hissing gurgling sound, as they gasp for air. They chase me, until I reach the top of the structure. That's when I realize there's nowhere else to go. I am trapped! The imps inch slowly forward; I can hear their awful sound. As I carefully move backwards, I suddenly slip and lose my balance. Now, everything appears in slow motion as I fall hundreds of feet. I look like a little rag doll bouncing and flipping off every pipe I hit. Falling down was very painful; I feel I had many broken bones. I tried desperately to grab on to the slippery pipes. I just could not hold on. Busted up and broken, I finally smashed on the concrete floor. The demons encircle me, rubbing their hands together with glee. I could hear the gurgling sound as I feel myself fade away. Crashing on the floor always seems to wake me up.

OUT OF BODY EXPERIENCES

Travel—Fully Awake—Jan. 01, 2002

While relaxed, sitting on a chair in my living room, I laid my head back and closed my eyes. This is what I saw in my mind. When I say that I see something in my mind, it is an actually running movie with both pictures and sound. My doctor calls them events. I have experienced this type of event many times in my life. I would call this some type of travel. My doctor tells me this is an out of body experience, induced by trauma. I remember when I was on restriction, as a child, I would be required to sit on a metal folding chair for hours. I had to do this many, many times so I knew what would happen. I learned that if I relaxed and let all of the pains in my body become numb, I could leave this location and travel to anywhere I wanted. I did not require any former knowledge of the destination. The locations would just come from my mind. This would happen all by itself. I was never afraid of these travels. I thought it was very cool, because the parents did not know anything about what was happening. I had a sense of being free from their overpowering control. At least for a short amount of time I was free. I was also on restriction for a period of two years. This happened the last two years I lived at home. During this time, I was only allowed to leave the basement, so that I could attend school. I used this two-year period to travel to many places.

I will try to explain the travel I went on this morning. It is the first day of the New Year—and no, I did not get drunk last night. I hope I can explain what happens so you can understand what this is like. I am not sure that the content of the journey is as significant, as the actual ability to travel itself. See what you think.

In my minds eye, I saw a black background. I sensed that I was moving upward. I began to see that I was in the air, above the earth. I was gracefully floating. Not like in a jet with speed, not like in a helicopter with spinning blades, or not like in a small plane with the sound a single engine motor. This is a soft gentle journey. I have a 360-degree view. This is all in color. I am above an old city with many buildings. None of the buildings indicates that this is a modern city. The buildings look like they are made of mortar of some type. The countryside is lush with vegetation. There are houses enough for thousands of people. I am high enough to see all over the countryside. I do not see little things like animals or people down there. I begin moving along at this height going slower and faster as I view the surroundings. As I travel, I turn away from the city. I can see a hill, and another very large hill coming up in front of me. There is a large mountain coming up so I have to rise above it. I can turn back and see the mountain behind me.

There is a wide river with some white water flowing below me. I am high enough to see this river between the hills. As I continue, I go over the next hill and see a low desert valley approaching. As I look to the horizon I see large rocky like structures reaching upwards from the desert floor. They appear dark, as I view the sun rising between the two great stones.

This travel went on for a long time. I will stop here. I think you get the idea. These experiences of travel do not give me any pain or sadness. I understand this is how the brain protects itself from trauma.

Travel In Tubes—Feb. 2, 2002

Yesterday a strange thing happened to me. This all happened in my mind while I was a wake. I was sitting in a chair, in the living room, watching a movie on the television. As always, I had my journal nearby. I wrote this down immediately after it happened. I think you'll see why, I missed the whole show.

My eyes were open. I lost all sense of time. I didn't see this in front of my eyes, but in my mind. The background turned black and florescent tubes appeared. These tubes are similar to the ones used for cable TV. The view was in 3D. The tubes were larger in the foreground and slop off smaller in the back. There are many tubes and all shades of color. The one I went down was florescent yellow. I travel down the tube at a good pace....I am writing this directly from my journal.

I have a very strong feeling not to write this event down at all. I guess it is fear about what doctors might think. I know normal people have a real problem believing different kinds of strange things, but I have seen many wild things. Information on these types of subjects is hard to find. Maybe I can help others that are also experiencing these things. I say this because, I wish my mother had said or written down something. Maybe I would be able to find some answer to these problems. My mother, as I remember, started acting quite strange when she was in her mid to late forties. I wondered a lot about this, but I didn't know what questions to ask. My wife helped to pointed out many things that seemed to be quite strange. Anyway, to cut a long story short, she died in 1993. I became ill in 1995; I was forty-four years old. More on this later, I thought I would just write this down while I had it on my mind. I should finish the story.

At the end of the tube, I was dropped off or landed in an unknown location. I would describe the place as a hall of halls. All of the walls had evenly spaced doors. This is hard to describe, but here goes. The place was not like a maze. All of the halls were of equal length. All of the halls connect to another hall. It appears from above to be divided up in to equal blocks. The wall covering was the color of red bricks. The doors and doorframes were all painted maroon.

I spent all of my time going up and down the halls. I tried to open every door. None of them would open. I discovered a very strange thing. There were no doorknobs on any of the doors. I went into a panic, because I could not find anyway out. I grew tired of searching the endless halls. With sweat on my brow, I turn left at the next corner. Rays of light were streaming across the floor startled me! The stained wood floor reflected the sunlight. It seemed warm and inviting as I looked down the hall. At the end of the hall, I saw a window. It looked like colored stained glass. It had a blue boarder and a triangle shape of regular glass in the center. My heart skipped a beat. Maybe I found a way out. I ran down the hall to the window as fast as I could. I peer out the window, feeling the warmth of the sun on my face. Then, I realize the window was frosted, I couldn't see a thing. I turned around with disappointment and hung my head down.

As I opened my eyes, I saw someone in the hall. I wasn't even shocked or scared. It was as if, in my heart, I knew that a little boy was sitting there. His back was towards me; I could not see his face. He was wearing denim overalls with a gray long sleeve shirt. I walk around him on the right. I notice his legs were up and he was resting his arms on his knees. His head was hanging down resting on his arms. His shirtsleeves were wet from his crying eyes. He never looked up at me. He never made a sound. The little boy acted as if I were not there. That's when I noticed; I was high above the hallway looking down.

After my wife read this story she said, it appears that the little boy was trapped. Maybe he's weeping, because no one hears his cry for help.

On Feb. 7, 2002, Dr. Wadeson read this story. He told me that this could very well be an out of body experience; because he said noting that, I was above the hallway looking down. We talked about this and other things at length. I discussed with him a possible meaning to this story.

I told him the halls could be the pathways of life. The doors are entrances to opportunity or answers about my illness. The fact that there are no doorknobs to open the doors may show that no solutions have been found. The warmth of the sunlight shows, that not all hope is lost. The frosted glass shows, that I have not found a direction in which to turn. "Could it be that I am the little boy?" In the story he is sad and crying, because no one could hear his cries for help. The fact that I am looking down upon the scene shows that I am having a very strong interest in what happens to this little boy. "Could this be the child within me?" As with most of the experiences like this, there is not always a cut and dry answer to everything in life. I will just keep searching for answers to these most troubling things.

3

What Are Intrusive Event Memories?

INTRUSIVE EVENT MEMORIES (IM)—DEC. 26, 2001

These memories are vivid intrusive movies. They are not like 35 mm slides or momentary flashbacks, which may last for a brief period. These event movies, as they are called, are running in my mind all the time. These intrusive event memories are just one of the other symptoms of PTSD. The event movies run twenty-four hours and seven days a week. I do not have to see, think, hear, smell, taste, or feel anything to start these intrusive event memories. Those I have listed above are called "triggers." A trigger may start memories, dreams, or feelings to occur in the brain. To complicate matters, there are from forty-six to fifty event movies all running in my mind at the same time. I am estimating the quantity of events running at one time, because when the number goes higher than this, I become frozen in a trance. While in a trance, I lose all sense of time and space. I'm in the past re-experiencing the trauma. I'm not aware of present time. I have found that a loud noise or some action that startles me suddenly will bring me out of the trance. The number of event movies running in my mind is then reduced to fifty or so. At which time, I become aware of my surroundings.

It must be emphasized, that these Intrusive Memories (IM) are not initiated, controlled, or stopped in anyway by the person having this occur in their mind. One terrifying part of having an IM experience occur is the total lost of control, which the person feels about the events happening, both inside the mind and physically outside the body. The viewing, content, duration, feelings, and re-experiencing the IM events are as if the trauma is happening again, in the present. When I first became ill, I was trying to explain to the doctors that I would become trapped in my own body. I had no control over my body. It's as if my mind had taken over, all by its self. I know now, after nine years of therapy, that this was an accurate description of what I was experiencing. However, I could not explain this to Dr. Wadeson adequately until recently.

My View of These Intrusive Event Memories—Dec. 26, 2001

I am not dreaming, hallucinating, or contriving these intrusive event memories. The event memories I view are not in front of my eyes. They are in my mind. I will try to describe how I view these events the best I can. If I may set up the backdrop, close your eyes and view a black background. Now, view one picture projected on the background like you would see on a television screen. View one additional picture inside the first picture. Continue adding more pictures until you are viewing fifty or so pictures all on the background. Continue until you cannot seem to add any more pictures. OK, at this point view all of the pictures changing size (all of the pictures are square). Now change all of these single pictures into running movies. Now, you can see that it is hard to describe the exact content of each event movie. I have a little help. Each of these event movies is about a trauma that occurred sometime in my life. I have been working for nine years to determine where, when, why, how about each of these intrusive event memories (IM). I am also trying to find out how to stop all of these intrusions on my mind. I had these questions on my mind. "When, will I begin to think about normal things again?" "When, if ever, will I be able to go on with my life?" This appears easier said than done.

As of this date Dec. 26, 2001, I will begin documenting all the information and subject matter about my (IM). My hope is that this information may help the doctors to find a solution if not a cure. To date, there is not cure for PTSD. IM's are just one part of PTSD.

This whole book has been part of my own recovery. This technique has a person write every detail of the traumatic events a person has experienced. This is a very painful technique, which forces the person to relive every moment of each trauma. During the review they will vividly see, feel, touch, smell, and experience all of the violence caused during each of the traumas.

This technique is call "imaging narrative writing." This is a rather new procedure, so the results are not in on its success rate. From my personal point of view, it has improved my mental state. It doesn't make the trauma go away; it helps you find your own way of dealing with the trauma. One MANDATORY

REQUIREMENT, while a person is undergoing this procedure is they must work with a Psychiatrist.

"NOTE: The DATES next to the headings are the actual dates I completed deciphering the (IM), and wrote the entry in my journal. I have placed the information in chronological order when I could.

Dr. Wadeson thought it would be educational to reveal both the time and energy required to complete this process. Within each section, I have left every emotional expression from my journal, so you can view what occurred to me as I relived each trauma."

CHILDHOOD ABUSE RELATED INTRUSIVE EVENT MEMORIES (IM)

The Fire (IM)—Trauma—Jan. 6, 2002

I knew my home life was not wonderful, but I never could tell exactly what was wrong. I was just a child. "What did I know about the great scheme of things?" I spent much time praying that things would get better. I always thought things should be better, nicer, and kinder than they were. "Why did life have to be so sad and cold for us kids?" Not all of the other children and their families seemed to have these kinds of problems. Our family seemed some how to be outside of the normal lines. I wished we were regular people!

This was my view as a child about to enter the third grade. At that time, I saw things in a very simple way. Parents can't fool us children for very long. Children seem to see through all the obstacles placed in their view. Finally, we got the news. We were getting a divorce!

Mom was leaving and we were staying with Dad. Then we were moved over to Mom's house. We did not think this was good or bad. The new house was nice as I remember. There was a yard and it had grapevines growing on a big trellis in the back. There were white benches attached to the trellis. This was going to be fun. It was nice sitting on the benches as the summer breeze blew through the vines. It was a cool area to just sit and enjoy the summer sun. Then, I remembered the fire!

My father came over to visit us kids. He was standing at the screen door on the front porch. We were told to go upstairs to our room. We ran as fast as we could up the steps, but we took a little detour and lined up on the top step. We wanted to hear what would happen. From the top of the steps, lying on our stomachs, we could see and hear everything. My father was still at the screen door and my mother was in the living room just below the steps. Yelling and arguing began and it was very loud. We crunched our little bodies and huddled tightly together. None of us made a sound. We could feel the tension in the air. All of a sudden, we saw it flying through the air! It was my mother's hot iron. We watched as the iron flew slowly across the living room. It tore right though the screen door. The iron landed with the hot side flat on my father's chest! I cannot remember what started the next set of yelling. I only remember words were flying as fast as the iron. The next thing I remember seeing my mother spreading newspapers all over the furniture in the living room. I heard someone say "Don't do that, stop, stop!" She lit the newspapers on fire! I could not believe my eyes! The smoke began to grow. It started coming up the steps. The smoke grew like a monster and filled the stairway. All of us kids ran, like a rocket, into the bedroom. We slammed the door and put the dresser in front of it! I was told by my older bother to get on the floor and watch for smoke coming under the door. While I was watching, my brother took out the window screen. He went out on the roof and I passed the kids to him. Then, I jumped into the tree. My brother passed me one kid at a time. I lowered each one down to the ground. We all ran to the backyard under the grapevines. We stayed there until a firefighter came to find us. One of my brothers said that he remembered my father coming to the back yard, but I don't remember it. I don't remember if the house burned down. The only thing I remember is we moved back with my father.

Punitive Correction (IM)—Child Abuse—Jan. 7, 2002

Most correction at our house was done with screaming, yelling, and beating with whatever was at hand to use. Intimidation, sadism, abuse, brutality, and absolute control were the normal course of events. Two weeks of restriction seemed to be the minimum restriction time for any type of infraction. There always seemed to be a reason to add an additional two weeks to a previous sentence. I didn't know anything about raising a family. I was a child. What did I know about how things should be?

I noticed that none of the other children, I talked to, were treated like us. I asked many questions, but never understood why we were treated badly! My parents were church going people. My father was a church deacon. They did not seem to do the things we had learned in church. Something was very wrong. I remember praying, at night in my bed, not to get beat tomorrow. This became a regular part of my prayers every night.

I am shaking and weeping, as I recount this story. Words cannot do justice to the emotions that I feel. No one cared enough to help us children. I know the neighbors heard our screams! Our windows were open. The police officer living in the house next door NEVER said a word! When our screams went unanswered, I saw them looking out windows and staring out doors. They NEVER said a word! The teachers at the school could see our ever-present body marks. They were patriotic, welts of red, lines of white, and bruises of blue and black. They NEVER said a word! Parents send their kids to church, so they will learn right from wrong. Parents send their kids to school, so they can learn how to do meaningful and productive work. Society wants each child to learn respect for each other and respect the law. These same people can't even help a screaming child! When I was a little child, all I wanted was a big person to help us. No one ever said a word! "What is wrong with this picture?" They NEVER said a word!

Let me tell you about a formal beating. This is different from being slapped in the head and knocked to the floor. This is different from a fist punch in the chest. This is definitely different from being yanked naked from the shower by my stepmother and beaten around the head and shoulders.

A formal beating is the process where the whole family assembles in the dinning room. We all line up by ages, on one side of the room. There's Dad, Stepmother, and five of us kids. All of us knew exactly how this was done.

This is very hard for me, that is, to put it down on paper. Children are never to tell what is happening in their home. It's as if all of the other dirty secrets people have in their minds and hope will never be revealed. "How can I express this?" I feel like a prisoner of war. There was no way out! I tried everyway I knew how to escape. As children, we would plot how to kill our parents! Then, we would be free. We didn't care about going to prison or anything else. It had to be done! It was that plain and simple. We talked about killing them for years. We were working out all of the details. If no one would help us get out of here. We would have to do it ourselves.

My stepmother would turn around a chair. The candidate would be instructed to drop their pants and shorts, and then bend over the chair. This was very humiliating to have done this to us in front of the whole family. In this case, I was the candidate. I remember when I bent over the chair. My pants were down upon my ankles. My toes just touched the floor. I can hear my belt buckle ringing on the floor as my legs shook with fear. I looked back to see what was in her hand. She yelled, "Turn around and put your head against the chair". She had ten; three-foot switches in her hand. I heard her screaming, "liar" with every downward stroke. She hit every place from my butt down to my ankles time after time. At times, she was jumping up into the air to make every downward stroke really count. The strikes were so forceful the switches began to break. I knew she would not stop until all the switches were broken into pieces. By this time, I was covered with red welts and blood. The pain I felt was so bad, it's impossible to explain. Sometimes it was so bad I hardly knew my name.

This happened to all of us kids many times. As I got older, I learned to control my pain. I was able to take a beating and not show any emotion. Not even, shed a tear. A deep hatred grew inside of me! I disconnected myself from almost every feeling. I got to the point that I felt no feelings at all. My stepmother got extremely angry, when I would respond with self-control. I felt satisfied, because I may not have controlled the events, but I sure controlled its outcome.

I have only recently learned about Dissociative Disorders (DD). The disconnecting of feelings is a natural occurrence. This is one of the ways that the mind protects the body. I did not know that disconnecting my feeling would cause any type of problem. I was just learning how to survive. I haven't learned how to turn my emotions back on yet. I have emotions going on inside, but I have forgotten how to let my feeling show. My wife says she can see emotions I have that others do not see.

One Thousand Times (IM)—Child Abuse—Jan. 7, 2002

When I was a child, we always went to church. All of the family sat together. We practically took up the whole row. Everyone stood up to sing a familiar song. For some reason I felt different that day. I did not feel like singing! I did not mean to be disrespectful. My mind was off in play land, day dreaming of things I would do. Boy was I wrong! I saw the look my stepmother gave me and I knew something was up. It was the, "Your in for it now, look!"

When I got home from church, she began to yell and scream. She said, "For not singing the song in church, my punishment would be to write the song a 1,000 times!" There were no other instructions for me to follow. She said, "I would write this song and do nothing else until it was finished!" The song has four verses and one chorus.

It was summer time and I was out of school. I spent all day, every day writing this song. About two weeks into this endeavor, she asked to see what I had completed. I thought I was doing pretty well. Not even, close! I was sitting at the little desk that faced the wall. I handed her a large pile of papers. Much to my surprise, she began yelling, screaming, and flinging papers everywhere! I said nothing. I showed no emotion. I did not want her to see that I was upset. I could not stop my body from shaking. I could not even remember if I was sitting or standing. I thought she was going to beat me to death. She continued to tell me all the things that were wrong. The song was written on good school paper…the format was wrong…the chorus was missing. She expended an immense amount energy telling me what trash it was. "Throw it way and start again," she screamed. "Write each verse and chorus together. Write it on unlined paper. "It better be straight and neat!" I can still hear the echo, as she stomped down the hall yelling, "1,000 times, 1,000 times!"

It took me three months to write this song a 1,000 times. I was not allowed to leave the desk. I was not allowed to play or have fun. I was only in the fourth grade. This song brings back bad memories. I guess it is understood; I never enjoy singing that song.

Goodnight (IM)—Child Abuse—Feb. 11, 2002

The stories in this section I wrote from my journal yesterday. I shook so bad, that I couldn't hold my pen on the paper. I felt so sick; I had to lie down for a few hours. My headache went away, but my stomach shook all through the night. "This morning as I'm typing in this information, I feel a little boy that's crying deep inside of me!" I'm so frustrated and outraged over the way we were treated as kids. I shake all over with anger thinking about all of these torturous events. I hope I have the ability when writing, to show both the hurt and the pain that we had to endure for so long. Moreover, for us kids, we never found an escape. I just wanted you to know, that it's as hard for me to write these stories down, as it is for you to read them.

My wife and I have always had dogs. Our dogs are treated better than I was as a child. We have love and consideration for our dogs. We train them with patience and understanding. When we teach them, we find a way to get them to respond. We have never beaten our dogs. Beating a dog will break his spirit and his drive to succeed. I think that continually abusing and beating children will break their spirit and ability for success.

My stepmother had a fetish about having all the children come and kiss her goodnight. It didn't even matter if we had just been beaten or yelled at for something we did wrong. It didn't matter what the mood or atmosphere was in the home. This goodnight thing was a required ritual.

Now, keep in mind there were four boys and one girl. My stepmother had a bunch of rules and one rule was that none of us was allowed to wear underwear beneath our pajamas. At that time, boy's pajamas had an open fly in the front. There were no snaps or buttons to close the fly. All of us boys had the same problem. We knew that we were not weird. As we walked or moved, our private parts would stick out. We would have to pull ourselves back in; this was both demeaning and embarrassing for us. We noticed that our stepmother had a thrilled or amused look on her face whenever this problem occurred.

We pleaded with my father asking for his help! We told him how our pajamas were to thin and that anyone could see right through. We told him about the problem with the fly. He said, "Nothing!" He didn't hear our cry for help! Each time something like this would occur to me, hatred and anger would grow larger inside of me. He said, "These were her rules and that they would stand." I estimate that I was in the fifth grade at the time.

On one occasion, she was in the bathroom taking a bath. We came and knocked on the door just to say goodnight and leave. No that's not how it went! She, to our amazement, told us to come in. We were old enough to know about personal privacy. I could not understand why she would ask us to come in.

Unbelievably, she was lying back with her arms one on each side of the tub. She had her right leg under the water and the left leg up on the side of the tub. Now, we had to lean over the tub to kiss her on the lips goodnight. I can tell you, even at my young age, there were not enough bubbles in that tub.

There was another time when goodnight was necessary. It's too gross to write down here. Let your imagination go and I'm sure you can think of what could happen? We did the knock on the door routine and she said come in. Anyway, let's just say she was sitting on the thrown. This goodnight thing went a little far! I don't think this is the way to teach proper etiquette.

Coffee over the Head (IM)—Child Abuse—Feb. 12, 2002

My stepmother and father had us bring them coffee wherever they were in the house. We felt that we were, "The Five Little Slaves." When we would pour coffee, we didn't know if it was hot or cold. We just poured them a mug and took it to them. What small child knows that the coffee pot turns itself off; no one ever told us. One day I brought them coffee; they said it was cold. Right there on the living room rug, they poured both cups over my head. She began yelling, "Clean this mess up." All I felt afterwards was a big drop in myself esteem. I felt worthless.

Household Chores (IM)—Child Abuse—Feb. 12, 2002

I know that it is a normal thing to have children help with chores around the house. I think there is also a right and wrong way of teaching this. I know it builds self-confidence and a sense of belonging. Let me explain what our chores were like.

I was nine years old, when I became in charge of the kids. Kind of like the official babysitter. If anyone stepped out of line and got in trouble, well, I was in trouble too. We kids did all of the chores around the house. That included washing and drying cloths out on a cloths line, vacuuming, dusting, cleaning floors, washing windows, scrubbing down the kitchen. I think you can see that we did it all. We were the little slaves. There was no playing, having fun, or just messing around. There wasn't enough time in the day to play. All we did was chores, study the bible, and do school homework.

I personally never learned how to play. My grandson is trying his best to teach me how to play. Bible study is a very complex subject, which even some adults never master. Why would you have a child study the Bible alone!

Each day I made the children's breakfast, lunch, and dinner. There was no eating between meals. If caught breaking almost any rule, would result in a terrible beating. That beating would be with a belt, strap, tree branch switches, or an electric extension cord.

Keep in mind we were just little kids. Let's talk about house cleaning. I moved and dusted every item I could find in the living room. Then I would dust all of the items on the mantel. It would always seem that I would miss something. Each time an assignment was completed we checked it off a list. My stepmother would inspect each job-completed everyday.

One day, when I finished dusting the living room, my stepmother began to do the white glove inspection. She put a white glove on her right hand and with a smug look on her face; she used her index finger to wipe across each item. She would check her finger after touching each item. When she found the least bit of dirt or dust, she would yell, "Filth—This is Filth!" Then, with a pushing swipe, she would smear the dirt on my face. As she continued, she smashed more dirt on my face. It was now mixing with tears and made mud marks on my face.

As time went on, I learned never to show any emotion! I had learned by watching her face that she received great pleasure from hurting me, in everyway she could! In time, my father joined in with the abuse. After he joined in, we had nowhere to turn for help!

A Summer Vacation—Child Abuse—Feb. 12, 2002

One summer my parents took us to Pennsylvania for a vacation at my step grandmother's house. This was a remote location with one road up the mountain. The one event I remember most was what my stepmother said after she dropped us off. She looked at us boys and said with a sneer, "Keep your dicks in your pants!" Keep in mind I was only thirteen years old. No one had even discussed the facts of life with me. In fact, at that point in my life I was appalled at what I heard! It was degrading and showed that they had no trust, what so ever in any of us. I thought, "Is this how church going people talk?" I had already learned about morals at church. I could have thought of a hundred better ways to get that point across.

Kicked In the Face—Child Abuse—Feb. 13, 2002

I remember back when I was sixteen years old. I was going into the tenth grade. I wanted to get out of church school. I was sick of it. I thought I had enough church indoctrination since the fourth grade. I had heard it all week in school and then again in church on the weekend. They told us repeatedly, how all of the people in the world were such terrible sinners. That people would surely lead us astray from the straight and narrow. They explained how those sinners would all die at the end of the world. I really wanted to know how wicked sinners were; or see for myself if this was true; or maybe this was just another one of their tricks. I just had an overwhelming need to see some sinners, up close, for myself!

The tenth grade was the first time I had the chance to see wickedness for myself. I guess my parents were a little upset with me after I ran away twice during the summer.

I went to public school and rode a real school bus for the first time in my life. I had always walked or rode in a van to school. I was truly excited about this new adventure! Everything was so different and new. I was also excited about taking mechanical drawing; they didn't have that class at the church school. I enjoyed all kinds of art and really did well in history and biology. As always, I kept my feeling hid. The one class I never enjoyed was gym. The marks on my body from all the beatings were exposed from the shorts we had to wear for gym. When I took a shower, they could see the marks from my neck down to my legs. I saw how the other kids stopped and stared. I also, heard the whispers and the things they said to each other, about what they saw. I felt very distressed about these things. "What could I do?" I just sucked the pain up inside and went on with my life. I think I've felt this way all of my life. I just used my standard technique, which was never show any feelings. I guess it worked, because no one ever challenged or confronted me.

I didn't think I was the kind of person anyone could like! Because of the way, I had been treated all through my childhood life. I was sure I could never be loved! Even the songs I heard about love on the radio, seemed like they were talking to others, not me.

Much to my surprise, I met a girl that year. We talked most of the time at the bus stop, before and after school. It was nice to have someone to tell the things that were happening to me. She was astonished by the stories I would tell. The one thing she did for me was actually listening to what I had to say.

Behind the house where we lived, was about an eighth of a mile square of woods. All of the neighborhood kids would play there. None of us knew who actually owned it. We even built a fort high in a tree. I was very familiar with all of the trails and paths that ran through the woods. All around the woods were the neighborhood streets. This was no isolated area.

It was on one of these side streets, next to the woods, where a school bus was usually parked. This was an open area, where all the kids would hang out after school and just talk. There were streetlights there, so even in the winter the kids could hang out. Even the younger kids could play street games.

One day this girl and I were leaning on the bus talking. That's when I leaned over and gave her a kiss. "Wouldn't you know it, at that same moment, my stepmother drove around the corner?" She was home from work early! I knew she had seen us, my heart stuck in my throat. I looked at the girl and she knew I had to go. I held onto my books and ran as fast as I could through the paths of the woods. I came out on the other side of the woods at our driveway. I was totally freaked out; my stepmother must have really flown, because the car was already in the driveway.

I went down the driveway as fast as I could. I entered the house from the door on the driveway side. The entrance was like a bi-level; there were six wooden steps up to the kitchen and ten wooden steps down to the basement. As I came in the door, my stepmother was standing on the kitchen landing. She began yelling, "Where the HHH have you been?" I began coming up the steps to the kitchen starting to explain. She yelled again, "Where the HHH were you?" I stopped on the steps and tried to reply, "Talking at the bus stop."

Then like a flash, she kicked me square in the face! I fell backward and smashed my back against the door. I leaned to the left to catch my balance and my books and papers went flying everywhere. I fell down the basement steps and hit my head on the concrete basement floor. I hurt everywhere! I felt dizzy from hitting my head on the way down. I lost track of what was going on for a minute. As I was getting up, trying to regain my senses. I remember her yelling down at me, with a sneer, "I saw you kissing that girl!" I thought to myself, "What was kissing also a sin?"

For kissing a girl, I was placed on two years of restriction. I was only allowed out of the basement (dungeon), to attend school. I swore then, that when I got out of this dungeon, I would never go back again!

As a footnote: In the year of 2000, I went to the doctor suffering from sleeping and breathing problems. At first, the doctor thought that this maybe a type of sleep apnea. Upon further research, he determined that I had a sever blockage in my nasal passage. I went into the hospital for surgery and the doctor fixed the problem. After the surgery, he explained to my wife and me that my nose must have been broken, when I was a child. I told him that my stepmother kicked me in the face when I was a child. He finished the thought for me saying, "Yes, that would do it!"

Parade Around the House—Child Abuse—Feb. 13, 2002

I'm not sure if I should label this section child abuse or stupidity! There were four boys in our house. I don't think it really matters how old we were. I believe it is the parent's job to teach their children to respect themselves and others. Can anyone explain to me why, my stepmother walked all around the house with skimpy shorts and just a bra? Ok, is this logical? Kissing a girl is a terrible thing! However, it is correct to run around the house, half-naked! All right, so its summer and it's very hot. Couldn't she ware a halter-top, instead of parading herself in front of us boys?

This was supposed to be a Christian home. At church, I hear a lot about: love, peace, forgiveness, mercy, understanding, being discrete, and goodness. At our house, I only learned about, hate, fear, anger, distain for children, cruelty, evil, punishment, intolerance, manipulation, and control. I wonder whom these parents thought they were fooling. We were kids, but we were not idiots!

Thoughts from the Abused—Feb. 13, 2002

All of these things have been bottled up inside me for many years. I call them the dirty family secrets that we were never allowed to tell. It wasn't that we didn't want to tell them; it was because no one would believe us! No one would lift a finger! See at that time people believed, what went on in that man's house was his own business! I wish people would just wake up. Maybe you can't change the world, but maybe you can change the life of one child. See, no one heard us when we cried out for help! No one got involved. It was like we were children standing in the middle of the street and no one helped us as a big truck ran us all down!

I've found it very strange that when someone speaks out about wrongs being committed, they become the object of others hate and abuse. People don't like to hear that something is terribly wrong. Haven't we learned about what abuse and hatred can do from history! The people I have come across over the years just don't stand up when they see something wrong! It's not happening to them. It's not something they believe will change their lives. They look the other way and this hate, abuse, and torture that continues every single day! I hope that people will become braver or our future will be might grim.

Hairy Legs—Child Abuse—Feb. 14, 2002

Here are a few other weird things that happened to us kids. None of the brothers was ever allowed in my sister's room. This was one of our stepmother's rules. I had a good relationship with my sister, so she never cared if I came to see her. None of us children was allowed to wear deodorant, after shave, or perfume. I never understood what the reasoning was behind this rule. I can say without reservation, that all of us boys really could have used more than just a touch.

Now, my sister was of the age where she should have been allowed to shave under her arms and on her legs. We talked about this many times. She hated to wear little white rolled down socks. She wasn't allowed to wear stockings either. I saw the other girls and they all wore stockings. She felt terrible and was extremely embarrassed over the way the boys and girls talked about her. They made it seem like she was a dirty person. They treated her like someone that didn't care about herself. They couldn't have been more wrong, but how would she explain this to them. I told her not to worry; I would help her find a solution. I didn't like to see her feeling so bad. It could be that we came up with this idea together; everyone knows how great minds work as a team. That doesn't really matter.

We decided to get two tweezers and we would work on this project together. We would have to work in secret when the parents were not around. So I made a rule, I would not do under arms that would be for her to do! She agreed. We started working on the first leg. I would get ready to pull out a hair on her leg, and then I'd look up at her face. I'd say ready, she would scrunch her eyes, and then I'd pull. She said that wasn't too bad, so we continued. After working for a few days, all of the hairs on her legs were gone. She remarked that she felt emotionally great! Now I felt bad, because I pulled out all of her hair. She finished her under arms. Now, she didn't feel so bad. This really helped herself esteem. Best of all the kids at school didn't call her, "Hairy Legs," anymore. Our parents never yelled at us, so I guess we got away with this caper.

Washing Dishes—Petty Rules—Feb. 19, 2002

This happened the same year I had to write the song a thousand times. When the kids would do the dishes after a meal, there would always be two of us scheduled to work together for two-week intervals. This all sounds normal, except there were as always too many rules. It seemed that everything we did came with a bunch of incomprehensible rules. It's as if our parents stayed awake late at night like two engineers designing the latest toy. Just to come up with these rules. When washing the dishes there would be no talking, joking, tomfoolery, arguing, simple doing nothing, but washing dishes. It seemed to me that every house chore was made to be as boring as possible.

We really didn't like all of these rules and we would go around them whenever we could. We thought life was supposed to be fun! Even in a bad situation, we tried to have fun. We knew if we were caught, we would have to pay dearly. We decided sometimes we just didn't think, we were kids, and frequently we just could not help ourselves.

One night my stepbrother and I were washing up the evening dishes. I was washing and he was drying them and putting them away. Well, we were joking around and he wanted to play a little game. I thought why not, a little fun wouldn't kill us. He explained the game to me. One person would move his hand, with their fingers spread open wide, left, and right over the counter as quickly as they could. The other person would try to stab a knife in between his fingers as they passed quickly by. I thought this game sounded a little dangerous. I didn't know the game was called chicken! I didn't want to appear as though I was a poor sport. I went along with his idea.

I went first; I started moving my right hand from one side to the other. Things seemed to be going ok. He stabbed the knife down and it stuck in the counter right between my fingers. I thought that was good. I started moving my hand left and right over the counter. Then he stabbed the knife down and stabbed me in between my knuckles. The blood was spraying on the counter and upon the cupboard. He grabbed a rag and put it over my hand, which was still stuck to the counter. I was about to scream bloody murder! When he tried to calm me down, saying you know we'll get into trouble. I knew that a beating hurt more than this so I gutted it up and didn't make a sound. He said in a soft voice, I'm going to pull the knife out, so hold on! As the knife came out, so did a lot more blood. I could feel my eyes getting burry; I guess he could see it too. He held me up against the counter. The pain in my hand shot right up my arm! We didn't want to get beat or go on restriction. We just did what we had to do to stop the bleeding. The wound went all the way through my hand. The cut between my knuckles was about a quarter of an inch on the top and an eighth of an inch on the bottom. I learned a valuable lesson that day and that was not to trust him.

Many Other Rules—Child Abuse—Feb. 19, 2002

There were many petty rules that were placed upon us as children. I would like to show a list of things that my parents told us were evil. If we did these things, we were evil too. Then, I would like to show the common everyday, practical life experiences we never had, because of these rules. I'll let you decide for yourself about the common sense or logic used by my parents.

The Rule was, do not have, or DO any of these things!
Cartoons—Cartoons would make us stupid.
Comic books—Comic books are full of meaningless fantasy stories.
Baseball cards—Baseball cards would cause us to worship men.
TV shows—TV shows depict all the evil people can do.
Movies—Movies depict all of the kinds of evil acts done in the world.
Playing—Idle hands are the devils workshop; we should be studying.
Playing games—Games make us waste valuable study time.

Now, I would like to show what I think can be gained using these valuable tools. I think my parents biggest mistake was never letting us just have fun.

Cartoons allow a child's mind to enter a time and space that will never be available to them again. They can dream anything. Anything is possible in the make believe world. This is a world where their thoughts and ideas grow as large as a big red dog that is bigger than a house. This is called having fun.

Comic books allow a child to travel to distant planet, galaxies, fantasy islands where pirates roam the high seas, image playing cops and robbers like Dick Tracy, imagination is exercised to untold limits, and ideas are planted in a child's mind of what could be. This is a time when they should be free of the have knowledge of all of the problem and complications in the world. They should be allowed to have fun enjoy childhood.

Baseball cards these cards open a child's mind up to the objective of memorization. When a child is young, it is hard to hold their concentration for ten or even fifteen minutes. Watching my grandson playing with cards, he spends a large about of resources learning names, batting averages, counts of home runs, and names of teams. As basic as this information is, this information will be the center of many a conversation. It's called trivia. I do not have the knowledge about any kind of trivia. This limits my social conversations. Again, the child is having fun.

TV shows these show both real and not so real life situations. A child should have a rich set of background knowledge about how life actually is. Children also learn about different ways to look both at themselves and at those around them. It is a child's depth of perception, which brings knowledge and new ideas to the forefront of their minds. This is a fun way to learn many different things; what's wrong with that?

Movies teach about all kinds of wonderful things. Many of the movies are shot on location. The movies bring travel, nature, science, history, and the universe directly to the fingertips of a child. Many of these things the child would not know if it were not for movies. Movies make learning fun. Children should have fun.

Playing is never a waste of time. Playing is the heart of socializing. All people must learn the skills to socialize to fit into the fabric of society. Even George Washington played marbles to relax. Without the knowledge of playing around, life becomes drudgery and a bore. Children should play and have fun.

Playing games helps a child understand how to: share, win, loose, kindness, courtesy, and understanding. They learn about competition, and we all know that's what life is about. So playing games for a child is essential for them to understand our world.

Cleaning the Kitchen—Child Abuse—Feb. 15, 2002

I always hated when Sunday came. This was another regular trauma day. Each Sunday one of us was assigned to clean the kitchen. The procedures in this story were performed the same way every weekend.

I remember that I was short enough to require a chair to reach upon the counter. Let me tell you what was required to clean the kitchen the proper way. The stove had to be cleaned both on the inside and out. The refrigerator had to be emptied and every article in it had to be washed and returned to its original place. All of the cupboards above and below the counter had to be emptied and every article in it had to be washed and returned to its original place. The window blind had to be taken down and washed. Then, the windows, walls, and floors had to be scrubbed. This took me over four hours to clean the kitchen.

Then, came the decisive moment, I placed a check on the board showing that the job had been completed. If my stepmother was in the house, we were required to announce that the job was done and ready for inspection. I really hated the part that came next.

She would enter the kitchen as if it were the first time she had ever seen this kitchen. Her eyes would scan the ceiling, walls, floor, counter, and the stove. If she found any grease or food on the stove, she would pick it up with her finger and smash it in my face. She would always yell, "Filth, this is filth." I could see by the expression on her face that she was going to enjoy this inspection. She rubbed her finger on the window ledge, counter corners, and back edges of everything. Saying her same favorite phrase again and again, while rubbing dirt, grease, food, dust, toast crumbs all over my face. If I had done well and she found nothing wrong, she would still get upset, because there was nothing for which she could yell. I knew I could not win at this game. I just waited for what she would do next.

Then she opened one of the top cupboards. She rubbed her finger over every can stored there, until finally three cans down she found dust. Bam, the dust went on my face. I showed no reaction at all. I stood as solid as a brick. Then, she would blow a fuse! She would start throwing everything out of the cupboards down on to the floor. I watched as flour mixed with a broken bottle of spaghetti sauce. The big cake she was creating on the floor just continued growing. The boxes of rice broke when they hit the pile, more cans, and bags of beans breaking all over the floor. The floor was a giant mess. Inside I was crying, yelling, and screaming saying, "What in the hell is all of this about!" A little dust was better than this mess. It made me so angry I could have killed her!

She had been screaming and yelling in a rage like a crazy person! Then she turned to me and screamed, "Clean this mess up!" as she walked out of the kitchen.

I always felt so helpless! Why was this happening to me? What did I ever do to deserve this? How long will I be able to take this? I longed to get away from this madness. None of this made any sense to me—It still doesn't make sense to me today. I prayed for help many times. I never understood why I couldn't receive just a little help.

Well, I repeated the cleaning process again. It was dark before I finished cleaning up the mess. The next time she came into inspect the kitchen, she just walked in, looked around and said with a sneer, "Ok, you can go to bed."

As I went down to my bedroom, I was dumbfounded. I didn't get it. What was all of this excitement and trouble suppose to teach me? I didn't win. I didn't loose. I didn't learn anything useful. I just think back over all of those wasted Sundays, I could have been having fun. I never learned anything constructive during my whole childhood.

Eat Like a Dog—Child Abuse—Feb. 17, 2002

This is a story that hurts me very much. One thing I've learned first hand about a family is that when one member is hurt, the other children feel the devastation.

The whole family attended for evening dinner. We were having spaghetti, salad, bread, and peas. My youngest brother was five or six years old. We were all eating. We were not allowed to speak much at the dinner table. The belief at the time was a child was to be seen and not heard.

My little brother dropped some peas from his fork. They rolled across the table and down to the floor. All of us kids thought it was neat how the peas went in-between everything on the table and never were stuck. We knew he hated peas, so we started joking and laughing, saying he was feeding the dog his peas.

Well, our laughter was short lived. Our stepmother began yelling again. This time it was all kinds of selective words about how sloppy could one person possibly be. She said my little brother ate like a dog and even worse than a dog. She went on to say that since you want to eat like a dog, we'd let you eat just like a dog.

With that said, she jumped up throwing her chair backwards. The chair turned over crashing on the floor. She grabbed up a hand full of newspapers and spread the sheets across the floor next to the wall. All this time she was screaming and yelling, now it was about, "You Pig," she grabbed the salad-serving bowl and dumped it all in the sink. Then she snatched up my little brother's plate and dumped it in the salad bowl. Still yelling she chopped and slopped everything together in the bowl. She threw the bowl splashing food on the wall as it hit the floor.

With a strong grab of his arm, she jerked him out of his seat and his chair went flying. Holding his arm, he was lifted through the air. He landed on the floor with the newspaper under his feet. She pushed him down on his hands and knees. Still screaming she sneered, "Now, go ahead and eat like a dog, and don't use your hands!!!"

These kinds of sadistic things were like a required trauma we had to experience on a daily basis. Yelling, screaming, loud destructive conduct, beatings, and demeaning act of all kinds were a regular occurrence in our home. As kids, I guess to cling to a little bit of sanity; we would joke with each other and say, "It's just another day at the Dorman house!"

Food Rationing—Child Abuse—Feb. 20, 2002

I was the child chosen to be both babysitter and cook. I was the child that made all the meals. I was the one chosen to enforce the rules pertaining to food allocation. I started this job at nine years old. Most people create appropriate portions for their children based on common sense. This was not true in our family!

Breakfast: When cooking hot cereal in the morning, I was only allowed to cook enough for one bowl of cereal for each child. There were to be no exceptions. If a child needed more food than allocated, he was labeled as a pig. Even if I could see that they were really, really, hungry I could not change to rule. This tore me up inside; I felt like I was responsible for starving my own brothers and sister. I knew this was wrong, so I would have to figure something out.

Lunch: The parents had another set of rules for lunch. When I made a cheese sandwich, only one slice of cheese was to be used. Each child only received one sandwich for lunch. It did not matter how hungry they were. If I made peanut butter and jelly sandwiches, I was instructed to scrape the excess off the bread. Our parents said that is so we do not waste the food. When I made lima bean sandwiches, which everyone hated I had to smash the beans, spread butter on the bread and scrape off what the parents said was wasted. Then, I would place a predetermine layer of beans on each sandwich. Again, only one sandwich was allowed for each child.

Dinner: Dinner was the same kind of story, so I won't bore you with the same details. I almost forgot. Each child received one plate of food. There was no such thing as getting seconds.

◆   ◆   ◆

I think it can be seen that these children were starving! With this kind of an environment where food is rationed, the kids would come to me saying their hungry. They would never think of going to or asking questions of our parents. All the kids were afraid of what might happen to them. The usual response from them was to get a beating. I thought they were just kids, and kids are always hungry. This was not a new concept. All parents with a half of a brain know this! Kids were like weeds! If you keep feeding the kids, guess what, they keep growing! I was a kid myself and this was a very big burden for me. I did not have a budget, with a set amount of money to buy food. I was old enough to have known, that if I went and asked my parents anything, especially to break one of the house rules, well they would beat the crap out of me. I knew we had to find our own solution. I felt that I was under constant pressure between the parents, the children, and all of the house chores that had to be done. I took on the challenge and did the best I could in a rotten situation. My stepbrother was treated differently than the rest of us. Our stepmother treated him like a normal kid. My oldest brother was thrown out of the house, by my stepmother, when he was sixteen. When we designed our master plans, there were secrets known only by my younger sister, two younger brothers, and myself. At this time, only four of the children were considered to be within this inside group.

Since all of us children were hungry, we had to find out how we could get food without being caught.

I made a secret plan that the four of us would stick together. I make up a few rules that would be easy to follow. We would collect all the money we found around the house while we were cleaning and put it in a jar. This was our special fund. The kids made up a list of all the can food that they liked. One of them was assigned the job of stealing a fork. Another kid had to steal a spoon. I took on the hard job of stealing a can opener. My bed in the basement was built into the wall, so our first place of storage for canned food would be under my bed box springs. The second place for can food storage would be down in the storm drain, behind the house, in the woods. The next thing we had to do was the actual stealing of the can food. I took on this job, because I knew when they went shopping for food and since I did the cooking, I knew what food was being used. The last thing we had to agree on was security. We could not have any wrapped or bagged items that would make noise. The other thing was we could not have our food storage areas invaded by bugs, which would surely give us away. We used the money to go across from the firehouse to a bakery called, "Gems Butter Gems." At the bakery, we could purchase a paper lunch bag of buttered dinner rolls for just three cents. We would always buy two bags. We would split them up four ways. The rule was that the lunch bags had to be placed in the outside trashcan. Since we put out the cans for trash pickup, no one would catch us. Everybody agreed on the rules, so our first plan went into effect.

This plan worked from the time I was around thirteen until I was almost seventeen and a half years old. That's about the time I moved out of the house. The kids did not go hungry for at least that period. For us, this was a good caper.

We watched closely how our plan worked and we made adjustments as we went along. We knew then, if we put our heads together, we could come up with a plan or caper as we called it, to overcome anything. Working together was good for us. For the first time we were beginning to have self-esteem. This gave us a feeling of strength over our situation. We had a special rule, which no one and that meant no one, would try to pull off something all by him or her selves. That could jeopardize any hope for our success!

The beatings were relentless! We knew no one would help us stop the beatings. So, we were determined to minimize them, as much as we could!

We worked like a little committee looking at each task to be done around the house. Not doing chores perfectly was the main cause of beatings. We decided that the kid that liked a certain job would be assigned that job. If no one liked to do a job, well tuff, you were volunteered, and were awarded the job anyway. We also, found out the differences and similarities for all of the work being done. Then, we set up a group of kids to do the work and another group to come behind them and do our own inspection, just as if our stepmother would do. This plan really worked and it helped us in two ways. This reduced the number of beatings for each person. Everyone was happy with those results! This plan gave us an added bonus, which we had not even imagined. We finished all the tasks more quickly, so now we had extra time to play! This was great we thought! We were like our own time management team, before we even knew what that was.

We made our own time to go out to play:

Going out to play was not that simple. We needed to make a plan in which we had all bases covered. The playtimes had to be coordinated. Everyone had to synchronize his or her watches. We had to make sure that no matter where you were or what you were doing—The time schedule had to be followed to the letter. We even used walkie-talkies to communicate an emergency or danger. This may sound like over kill, but when the parents called on the phone or if they came home early. We had everything covered and we never were caught. See to us none of these things were classified as dishonest. This was survival. We had to do these thing to try to live what we thought was a normal existence. We knew we were dealing with a terrible problem, because none of the kids in the neighborhood had to do these things just to be a normal kid.

The parents watched TV in their bedroom. Why would they do this if it were such a sin? We decided to make a plan, by which we could watch TV, and not are caught! Again, to make this work, we had to collect information. We worked out every detail about our parent's comings and goings. How long they stayed at work and the exact time each of them got. We charted this everyday of the week. Then we had to remember what days were holidays or vacation. We checked their room everyday and noted where every item had been placed. We always checked the window blinds to ensure correct positioning. We noted where any pieces of clothing were placed. We checked the positioning of the throw rugs and if there were footprints on them. We checked the lighting if lamps were on or off. We even noted where the empty outlets were. Now, the most important subject to analyze was the TV. What channel was it on; we had to remember the exact positioning of the antenna. We had to find out if the cord was plugged in or not. We found that they took the TV electric cord with them when they left. We went and bought an electric cord that could be used with the TV. We made up rules of conduct; responsibilities each child was in charge of ensuring things were the same when we entered as when we left. One kid had a flashlight, instructed to point it toward the floor. It was only turned on as exited the room. Someone was in charge of looking out the window, to see when a car would pull in the driveway. Another one was in charge of décor. That is making sure everything we had discussed was in its exact place.

We rehearsed all of the procedures, until we had them all down pat. Again, we were successful and we were able to watch TV for the first time. We watched shows like Mc Hales Navy, Lost in Space, and our favorite Mission Impossible. When the parent came home all that would be seen in the room was kids moving at lightning speed. Everything was done with precision. We had some narrow escapes, but we never were caught. After restoring the room, we would fly to our bedrooms. Of course, we were fast asleep when the parents came in.

A Little Aside From the Thoughts of the Kids

As children our belief in ourselves, in our ability to overcome the odds was very important. We believed that it was us again them, the parents. We were like a little army fighting against a foe. We learned from Mission Impossible and other spy shows that every detail had to be planned and tested. We spent many hours working out our plans. We rehearsed them down to a 'T'. We did this all with our stepbrother in our midst. We just told him that if he said anything, then we would just have to tell the parents about him and his girl friends. That solved that problem quite well. I hope it does not sound like we were bad devious kids, because I don't think we were. We did things to make our lives better and we didn't approve of hurting anyone.

We thought we were doing what we had to do in a hostile environment. The people that lived around us were quite aware of everything that went on. Everyone knows how much information a nosey neighbor can pick up. Believe me they knew. Then we had to deal with the convention, "A mans home is his castle". Well, how about the convention we saw in effect, "A mans home is his cesspool."

Did anyone consider the crap we had to go through! I can remember the wonderful women from the church they had beautiful perfume on, they would put their noses so high in the air, that if a rainstorm came they would have surely drown. Yes, we knew about church people they had such caring hearts, if we asked for help they would say we would love to but…. it's very complicated, you children would not understand. Right! Yep, we understood, we knew a lot. We could even see that BS must be very heavy, because it ran down hill very fast. Everyone had concern, that is, concern for his or her own. No one had time to reach out to the little Dorman kids. To see if something was wrong or how they could help? No, but they had time to support starving children half way around the world. No one wanted to get his or her fingers dirty exposing apparent evidence against one of their own. This was the first time I learned about the "Old boys club." Of course, I didn't know the name of it, but I could see what they said and that was they had to take care of one of our own.

Knife by his Head—Child Abuse—Feb. 15, 2002

I had become increasingly enraged about the circumstances in which I was living. One might say I was on the edge of blowing my stack. I was in my second year of restriction that had totally overwhelmed me! I had been placing an "X," on my calendar each day as it passed; I knew exactly how much time I had left to stay in this hellhole. By this time, I hardly spoke at all to my parents, even if they were talking directly to me. I wanted them to try hitting me again or even getting me pissed. I was ready to lash out and kill either of them! I didn't care or even have any concern about what might happen to me. My anger was now at such a point they could probably see the flames coming out of my eyes. My level of hate was so great; I knew my stepmother could feel it as I walked by. I was just waiting for any opportunity to strike out. Being on restriction for so long, taught me the ability of self-control. I felt like a wolf waiting for the first stupid rabbit to stick out his head. These words do not show the amount of rage that I had bottle up inside of me. I had time to contemplate all the abuse and torture I had endured, for almost nine years. I had nothing, but contempt for my parents. As I came home from school that day, I entered the house by the side door; I heard a thumping sound. I was standing on the entrance landing below the kitchen. I looked up the six steps to the kitchen door. I thought that door was normally opened, but it was surprisingly closed. I still heard the curious thumping sound. I slowly went up the steps, listening as I went. I entered the kitchen to find my younger brother being held up against the wall by my father. His feet were not even touching the floor. The thumping I heard was the sound of my father pounding him in the chest.

Well, I lost it! I grabbed my father by the shoulder and pulled him backwards, with all my strength. Bam, he hit the floor with a mighty thud. He appeared stunned and surprised. I quickly scanned the counter for any object I could use for defense. I pulled the largest butcher knife out of the stand. I jumped down on the top of his chest. His arms were out at his sides. As he moved his arms down, I blocked them with my legs. I grabbed him by the throat with my left hand; I was holding the knife in my right. I quickly raised the knife above my head. I looked him dead in the eyes! Frozen he didn't move a muscle!

In my mind, I was thinking where and how hard I should plunge the knife. As I looked into his face, I saw his eyes go blank. I made my decision and down came the knife with all of my strength. I stuck the knife into the kitchen floor about a half an inch from his right side of his head.

I got off his chest and I stared deep into his eyes as I screamed at the top of my lungs, "If you ever beat him like that again, I won't be sticking the knife in the floor the next time!!" I glanced over at my brother and gave him a wink. I walked out of the kitchen and went to my bedroom in the basement. This event has never been talked about or ever discussed again. I guess this shows that even domesticated animals, like children, will kill!

Trip Away To Florida—Early Release—Feb. 15, 2002

During the tenth grade, I made a plan to run away and go to Miami, Florida. It seemed like a long distance to me in those days. Half of the school kids said I shouldn't go. The other half bet me that I would chicken out and be too afraid to go. It didn't matter to me what anyone thought. I was sick of it; I had my mind made up. Look out Florida here I come.

I was still living with my father and stepmother. Nothing had changed. They still beat on me every chance they could. I didn't really care about what they would do when I returned from the trip. I had already been on restriction for a year, what did I have to lose? I still had another year of restriction to go. In a year, I would be 18 years old; there was no law that would keep me from leaving. No one could change my mind.

In June of that year, I purchased a round trip ticket on a Trailways bus from Washington, D.C. to Miami, Florida. I earned the sixty dollars cutting peoples lawns. I had a few extra bucks, just for spending money. I wasn't broke. I wasn't worried or scared about anything that could happen. Since I was young, I didn't think of those types of things. All I saw in my hand was a, 'get out of jail free' ticket. I was going to use that ticket as fast as I could. It wasn't everyday that I could break out of prison.

I sat patiently in the bus terminal. I wasn't even bored. I wasn't in a hurry; I'd get there soon enough. I thought it quite funny, listening to the conductor call out the destinations of the cities where the buses were headed. He called out in a deep voice, "Fayetteville, Charlottes Ville, Pools Ville, and Jacksonville." He would just go on and on, rhyming names of cities. I thought he sounded funny, but from his voice, I could tell he enjoyed it. I had taken history in school, but I never noticed how many Ville's they had down south.

All I could think was, "I was free!" I thought to myself, that I could do most anything, and not even get beaten. This was like a dream come true. I thought wouldn't it be strange, if this was my way out! Oh! What a dreamer I was, now that I look back on those youthful times. I continued thinking; I would be going through five states heading south to Florida. This was a great idea; I was thrilled; I knew I'd enjoy the whole trip! I felt, maybe for the first time in years, I FELT excitement coming from way down inside me! This trip was really a good thing! My bus was scheduled to leave that night; I had the whole day to watch the different people. This was really the first time I had ever been away from home. There were people of all different colors and the cloths they wore, well frankly, they wore cloths I had never seen before. I saw rich folks; they were the ones that had someone else carrying their bags. There were normal folks; they all looked about the same. Then I saw for the first time people that were poor. They wore cloths that didn't match the weather and they carried grocery bags of stuff. I watched them for quite a while; I could tell they were poor; they never got on a bus. They just kind of hung around and people would give them money.

I never lost my focus; I was always listening for the conductor to call "Miami." Again, I thought, it really didn't matter what state a person was going to, if you didn't know the destination city; well, a person would be just sitting there after everyone else was gone. Yep! I'll just wait to hear, "Miami boarding on track 4." I really didn't know what a track number was; I just acted as if I knew what I was doing and followed the other people out the back door. I was glad they had all the buses facing toward us; I walked along in front of the buses and just by luck, there it was up on the front of the bus a big sign that read, "Miami." As I got to the bus, I must say I was relieved. I could have gotten on the wrong bus and ended up in California!

When I approached the bus, I noticed that there was a giant window in the front on the passenger's side. I must have gotten to the bus quickly, because that seat had not been taken. I thought to myself, that was my spot; my name was written all over it. I jumped in the front passenger seat quickly and made it my home. I knew that I would not miss a thing. With this big window, nothing would get passed me. I thought this is so great; I've gotten away! I knew I would have to control my excitement. I surely could not let it all out; that was a fact, they would have thrown me off the bus for being some kind of a nut.

There was a lot of talking chatter between the passengers as they chose their seats and settled in with their luggage. Everything got very quiet, when the bus driver explained some things over the intercom. I was extremely excited; I think I missed everything he had said. The lights dimmed a little and I heard a Ding, Ding. I looked about and noticed that we were pulling out from the bus station.

My great adventure had now begun! I noticed that there were no young adults my age on this bus. Everyone seemed to settle down for a long winters nap. I couldn't, there were a million thoughts going through my head. I thought I'd wait until we were out of the city. Then, I'd wait until we were going down the highway. Finally, I'd make sure there wasn't much traffic and then I would begin to speak. I felt sure that the driver would not mind, since everyone else was going to sleep. At last I could speak! I began discussing pleasantries with the driver. He understood how excited I was taking my first trip. He told me this trip, with all the stops, would take eighteen to twenty hours. I didn't think that was much; I've had to sit on my hands longer than that. The trip sounded to me like it would be a breeze. I eased back in my chair, but I never went to sleep. I didn't want to miss a thing. We made a few stops that night. It was great to see all of the different towns. Everything looked new and different to me.

Early in the morning as the sun was coming up, we stopped somewhere in South Carolina or Georgia. Everyone got off the bus and we went into the dinner. After talking during the night, the driver and I were friends. I went into the dinner and sat down with him. Now, I was a northern city boy. I never heard how southern people talk. I never went out to a southern restaurant in my life. I didn't know there were southern nicknames for food. Like the word grits. "What in the world were grits anyway?" The only grit I knew of was to grit my teeth. He looked at me funny, he was really enjoying this; I smiled, but had no idea what was going to happen. I kind of shrugged it off and picked up a menu. He asked, "Boy, what cha haven?" I pulled my menu down, looked right at him, and asked him why he was talking funny? He just laughed, but he didn't say anything more. I continued to look at the menu. Then I noticed that I couldn't read many of the southern nicknames on the menu. Well, I could read it of course. I just didn't know what the words meant. What is this France? Without trying to be a nuisance, I asked the bus driver in a low voice, "Can you read this stuff?"

He laughed and said to me, "Are you hungry?"

I said, "Yes!"

He said, "Are you really hungry?" I thought, this could go on forever and I am hungry. This time, I just rolled my eyes at him. I guess he got the message, because when the waiter came to take our order, he told her what we both wanted. I told him things felt a little strange here. These people seem to too friendly. They act as if they know us. He said, "You in the country now boy. They talk and act different down here." I asked him if the people in Florida spoke city English. He laughed at me and assured me they did. After eating, we all piled back on the bus. I guess one could say, the bus headed down yonder, a ways.

When I arrived in Miami, Florida, I went and checked into the YMCA. It was a nice place and it didn't cost very much. I swam in the swimming pool and worked out a little in the weight room. I felt much better after sitting on that bus for all those hours. This was my first day in Miami; the weather was nice and warm.

A teenager staying at the YMCA and I talked a little about where we were from. He said he was on his way out, but he told me to be sure and go inside a building around four o'clock each afternoon. "Why?" He said, "Because it rains!" I heard what he had said, but it didn't sink in. I just made a mental note of it waved and said thanks, as he bolted from the building. Being tired from the trip, I went up to catch a nap. I didn't wake up until the next morning. Probably I should have slept on the bus.

The following day I laid back on my bed gazing out the window. The blinds were closed, but the strong sun was shinning through. I thought that I'd go site seeing. Before I left, I thought I'd go up on the roof area to have a look around and write a letter. I sat on a bench with my side to the sun. It wasn't a very long letter; it only took me fifteen minutes to finish it. I felt like I was getting very warm, so I headed down to my room.

Much to my surprise the door to my room was opened! I knew I had locked the door before I left. I went into the room and looked around in a quick scanning motion. Everything I had with me was gone! My radio, suitcase, cloths, and even my cash money were all gone! I had been robbed! I went down to the desk to tell the manager what had happened. He told me how sorry he was and then he called the police. Everyone was quite nice to me, both the police and the YMCA manager.

The one thing I had left in my pocket was my round trip ticket back home. I thought, this is terrible, here I am away from home for only two days, and my dream trip was over. I felt like there was a black cloud hanging over me. Everything I try to do seems to backfire on me. I would not go home in disgrace! Maybe I could figure something out. I had paid for the room for a couple days. I had at least that long to come up with a new plan. After the police took down all of the information for their report, the officer said again he was sorry. He ended his conversation saying, that's the breaks kid.

I went back up to my room, laid on the bed staring at the ceiling. My heart was still pounding from all of the excitement. I just learned about how bad the tropical sun can burn a person with fair skin. I was half-white and half-Indian. I left the door open. I couldn't think of any reason to close it, the only thing left to steal was the sheet. I was feeling low. I must have dosed off a little. I was awakened, when I heard a knock on the door. I opened my eyes and standing in the door way was the teenage boy I talked to earlier. He said that he had heard what happened and asked what I was going to do. I told him I wasn't sure. Then he came up with a suggestion. "Why don't you come with me and I'll show you what I do?" I thought that would be ok, since I haven't figured anything out yet.

Well, he was street smart and he said he'd show me the ropes. With no money, he took me to a few burger shops. There we swept and mopped the floors for burgers and fries. The owner was very kind to us; he even gave us a coke too. I was in Florida only a few days. He showed me about the four o'clock rain. He said, "It's getting close to four o'clock we better get inside." I didn't have a clue of what he was speaking. Boy, did I learn fast. We were in a burger shop sitting in a booth. Just as he said, "It started to rain!" I thought to myself, he knew a lot from his experiences.

It didn't just sprinkle, nor did it just rain; I'm talking buckets of water were pouring out of the sky. Then as fast as the rain started, it stopped. The sun came out and all of the people came back out on the street. Everyone went about his or her business as if nothing had happened. He said, "It always happened just like that." It wasn't but thirty minutes later everything was dry. I saw this happen a few times before I left Miami. Like clockwork each day, we would make our rounds to the burger shops and we never went without food.

I had to tell my friend goodbye at the bus station. With my round trip ticket in my hand, I boarded the bus headed for home. As I made the trip home, everything seemed much different now. I knew that surviving in this world took a lot more cunning and experience than I had. I would have to think more about this as time went on.

Now, the trip home seemed to be dismal and gray. All the glitter, excitement, and thrill I had felt, had faded away. It didn't matter that the sun was shinning brightly through the window. It was the whole sense of who I was and what I had the ability to change that seemed different. There seemed to be many things in life, which I would have no control over. This really troubled me, because I guess for the first time, I realized that the things my parents were doing to us, would influence us for the rest of our lives. Thinking of this idea caused a light to go on in my head. This fact and the realization of this idea, was really going straight into my brain. I was realizing something, which I had never known before. This idea was not even in my mind, when I started out on this trip. Maybe this was a part of growing up that I was experiencing as I rode home on the bus. When I returned home, my stepmother was more than mad, she was flaming. My father was standing there, but he said nothing. I just gave them a cold shoulder. I didn't care about anything she had to say. I just went down to my bedroom in the basement. It was surprising though, they never said very much about my trip.

A couple of weeks later a letter came to the house from the Miami, Florida Police. They apologized for me being robbed, losing all of my belonging, and a few other pleasantries. My parents read the letter to me; they asked, what was the meaning of the letter? I saw the gleam in my stepmother's eye as though she had just uncovered a sinister plot. I didn't want to give her any information to help her figure out this mystery. I just said smuggle it was nothing, just standard questioning. I left it at that. Boy, were they confused. They really wanted to know all about the trip. Was I scared? Did I have fun? They were looking for anything that would prove to them that I had a bad experience. They always enjoyed seeing someone experience pain. I wasn't about to tell them anything. I was laughing inside; let them determine the answer of this one!

Away To Mother's House—Feb. 16, 2002

I made a plan to run away and go to my birth mothers house. I had to leave! I called her and arranged, where, and when to pick me up. It was June and school was out. She lived in a different city and county than I did. It would not be legal for her to cross a county line to pick me up. I told her I knew where the county line was located. She could pick me up at the movie theater. She agreed and we setup the date and time.

It was time for me to go. I had set up our meeting so that the parents would be at work. When I arrived at the theater, she was waiting for me. I got in the car and we sped away. We traveled a long distance to the other city. We talked about how I was doing, how was school, and about me living at her house from now on. I was glad; I thought this might be my way out of this life of torture.

Let me tell you a little background. My older brother was one and a half years older than I was. My father was sent to South Korea for a one-year tour. During that time my older brother became fed up with the torture and abuse, my stepmother put us through. One day as my stepmother was pounding on one of the kids; he stepped in and knocked her to the floor. My stepmother blew up and told him to leave. He was sixteen years old. The following day when he came home, he found everything he owned thrown out in the middle of the driveway. He just packed his stuff in a taxi and went to live with a friend. He stayed there for a year and during that time, he found out where our mother lived. I think it was after the school year he moved to my birth mothers house. When my older brother left, my heart inside of me was crushed beyond any words I can say! That was like the biggest loss I had ever experienced!

I had just lost the only big brother I had to protect me! I seemed to spend all of these years praying for help! "Why wouldn't God hear me?" "Again, and again, I would cry out for help!" I knew he saw everything that was going on! "Why wouldn't he help us?" We were just little kids. Didn't he hear little kid's prayers? That was when a huge uncontrollable rage, began to grow inside of me! There was nothing in the world that would stop this ragging fire contained inside of me! I decided that these people would have to pay—I didn't know how or when, but someday they were going to pay for all the torture they we experienced! I believed that inside I felt my situation was hopeless. As I understand the definition of the word hopeless, is to be without hope. I had nothing to hope for; to have any hope meant, I had to have something to look forward to; I had nothing, nothing, except more torture as far as I could see. Even today, I have this same rage, which burns inside of me! This is so upsetting to me; I am shaking all over and feel like I could explode! I'm going to go and lie down for a while. I can't write anymore write now.—Well, I slept for a couple hours and I have now calmed down. Sorry for the interruption, I'll go on with the story now.

My older brother discovered where my mother lived a few years before. He had moved there from his friend's house, after my stepmother threw him out. It was obvious to me that my birth mother knew everything about what was happening to us. When she picked me up, my birth mother told me that she was not legally allowed to take or visit us children. I heard what she said, but I thought considering all of the abuse we were going through, something should have been done. I have always pondered these questions and I don't think I was being told the whole story. I didn't say anything more about this subject as we drove to her house.

Once we arrived at her house, my older brother and I went to play pool. I had never been to a pool hall before. I felt great! I didn't know playing pool was that much fun! We ate lunch at the house and to my surprise; I could eat all I wanted! Back at my house, our food was rationed. This was like a dream come true! I felt that it might be good, if I could stay here forever. Well afternoon turned into evening and down went the setting sun.

Then the phone rang, I could tell something was wrong! My heart dropped! After the conversation was over, I remembered she said that was your father and he's coming to get you. It was as if hell had just opened and I was falling in!

My father had previously told me he didn't know where she lived. He didn't know how to reach her. Bull, everything he had told me was a lie! All these years he knew exactly where she lived; he just wanted us to stay with him. It didn't matter to him that our stepmother and he were beating the crap out of us everyday. I knew then, he didn't really care about the welfare of any of us kids! I personally do not understand the logic being used for any of the decisions he made. I could not help it; I just started to cry! Again, I felt there was no one that could help me.

In a few hours, my father arrived. I remember I was still crying and sobbing, while I explained the things they did to me. I pleaded for help! My birth mothers told my father, "Can't you see he's terrified? Nothing seemed to matter; I was doomed! I didn't want to go back home with my father. They had a conversation, but nothing seemed to make sense to me anymore. I felt like I was floating in space. The pain, fear, and anguish seemed to be held a short distance from me. I felt completely alone. I thought what I was experiencing was no life for a kid. None of these people seemed to understand the depth of pain I was going through!

The whole conversation was too complicated for me to understand. They talked about the past, about this thing that happened, and you did that. I thought where in the hell did I fit in any of this! Then they finally started speaking words I could understand.

My birth mother said, that I would have to go back home with my father. She said she had no other choice. She promised, if they beat me ever again, that I was to pick up the phone and call her. She would come and pick me up. She said when I was eighteen years old; I could come and live with her, but not before. My heart sunk low in my chest. I could tell by the look on everyone's face that these decisions were final. There was nothing to be said. I said my goodbyes, turned and walked down to the car.

I knew I was going to the car, but I could not feel my body. I was numb all over. I felt like the walking dead. Nothing seemed to matter. I sat in the back seat of my father's car, but I don't remember hearing anything on the long trip home.

The actions depicted in the above paragraph, I've learned through therapy they are called Dissociative Disorders (DD). The way the brain protects itself from an overwhelming load from anguish, torture, and despair is to disconnect the nervous system from the body. In this way, the brain stops the feelings at the source, therefore reducing emotions that would overwhelm the mind.

VIETNAM WAR COMBAT RELATED INTRUSIVE EVENT MEMORIES (IM)

The First Attack (IM)—Vietnam—Jan. 19, 2002

In June of 1968, I graduated from high school. In August, I was in the Navy boot camp and by December 1968, I experienced my first attack. The Vietnam War currently fought on all fronts land, air, and sea provided a graphic array of munitions. I learned a lot history about this war during my first year. I learned from people that had been there. Somehow, the story was very different from the one I'd heard at home. None of this did I consider? I was trained to do a job; that was the only thing on my mind.

The first day of the war for me, I never will forget. It was late 1968. When I close my eyes, I see myself standing at an open hatch.

We had just come from refueling, taking on food, and arms at another location. We were on a heightened status, so we were all on alert. We worked twelve hours on and twelve hours off. In the Navy, they call this type of working port and starboard watches. Besides the twelve hours work at a duty station, we were required to stand a four-hour watch. Everyone was working sixteen hours each day. It takes a while to get used to it.

From the open hatch, my friends, and I could see land on the left. It looked like we were cruising at about twenty knots or so. The sun had already risen; we could see the coast of Vietnam a few thousand yards away.

The ping, ping, ping of small arms fire was streaking across the deck. Then the sound to general quarters started ringing in our ears. I heard this sound in boot camp, but somehow this time it sounded more sincere. Men were flying, jumping, and running all over the ship. It was like watching a ballet, but no one wore tights. Protective gear was jingling; the smell of fresh rubber was everywhere. Then the turrets buzzer began the sounding off 1, 2, and 3, fire. The ship shook from the front, and then pushed up to the left. Another turret fired from back and we twisted to the right. They didn't show us this in boot camp, I thought to myself. Now, all the guns began firing to the beat of a different drum. The air had a distinctive smell of gunpowder. Flames shot out the barrels. Those were the loudest sounds I have ever heard. There was a mighty whooshing sound as the projectiles sped on their way. The ship was shaking violently. The ship seemed to be twisting underneath my feet. I could see that my fellow sailors were feeling the same as me. I could see the look in their eyes. No one said a word. Heads were shaking, and then their heads would bow. What a mighty force was unleashed on that day. The power we saw that morning brought us to our knees. I could not imagine what an atom bomb would do. I couldn't help thinking about the people where the shells would land. Since I was a radioman, I went up near the bridge. Looking out across the land, I saw the distance plums of smoke. I guess I saw the face of war that day and looked it in the eye. It's something no one can forget. It has taken me years to express what I have seen. A compassionate person is not a coward; he just knows when to quit. If someone says there's no fear in war, the person has probably never been there. They're not telling the truth.

The Mountain (IM)—Feb. 5, 2002

We were on the "Gun Line," that's what the Navy called the coastline 15,000 yards off the coast of South Vietnam. The year was 1968. I became 20 years old that summer. As we cruised along the coast of Vietnam, the climate always seemed to be summer and sticky. This country only had two seasons. One was hot and wet; the other was just plain hot. My job in the Navy was radio telecommunications. I was known as a radioman. The radio shack was one of the hubs of activity on the ship. Not to bore you with the details, but I was in a position where I could observe the planning, preparation, and execution of war activities. I have never discussed my work, so I will leave it at that. I just wanted to show you where my observations come from.

I was onboard the U.S.S. Newport News, the biggest heavy cruiser in the world during that time. Our sisters ship the U.S.S. New Jersey was the biggest battle ship in the world. What a great team the two ships made cruising along with a complete task force of ships. I remember watching the young men preparing for the events that would follow. Having one of these large 2,700 pound shells land on you was like having an exploding Volts Wagon dropped on your head. The New Jersey had many turrets, three barrels on each. The Newport News had many guns also. Having these two ships shooting at the same time shakes the earth and displaces the water around them.

One of the missions we went on was quite memorable. We received our instructions and began cruising towards our target. We were going around 20 knots. As a radioman, an enumerable number of visits were required up to the bridge, flag plot, and CIC delivering messages directly to the officers for signature. This made regular message rounds appear quite simple. The activity was very intense within every division on the ship, such as the bridge, radio, radar, and fire control. The preparations were rapidly underway; I was at attention on the bridge awaiting further instruction.

Without warning, all of the huge speakers sounded loudly. "General Quarters started to sound!!!" "General Quarter, General Quarter!!! This is not a drill!!!" "This is not a drill!!!" This sound, to a sailor, means to ready for an imminent attack. This is the highest call to readiness. The sound echoes everywhere, it's as if I were immersed in the warning! The alert went down my spine and though my whole body! I start telling myself this is it!!! We have come halfway around the world. Through endless training drills every division on the ship shaved second of their readiness times. Still standing at attention one the bridge I could clearly hear each division within the ship reporting readiness. We're ready! This was one of those times where thirty seconds, feels like a lifetime.

Everything became quiet, if that were possible under such conditions. Now, we await further instructions. It's like having your finger on the trigger of a huge shotgun. Nothing was heard, except commands and responses. The tones of all voices were different from before. The adrenaline was pumping. Everyone is at the peak of alertness. The air is thick with tension. Everyone knows what happens next. No one utters a word about what feelings are racing through their bodies. All of us could see the mystical ball was hanging in midair, all eyes fixed on the object, waiting for it to fall. Time stood still. It's the last second before we can stop this event from thrashing the earth. We heard no reprieve. The hour had come!

The Captain issue his order, "FIRE!" Every turret warning alarm went off. Buzz, buzz, buzz, and FIRE!!! All guns on both ships began to fire at once. The flames shot out for than fifty feet from the barrel of each gun. Followed by the inevitable sound, the shaking was indescribable. I thought the ship was going to fall apart from beneath my feet. Training allowed us to become accustomed to the sites and sounds of battle conditions. There is no training on earth, which can prepare a soldier for true combat conditions. Training can only be a small simulation. Never have I seen anything close, to the amount of raw savage power unleashed before us that day. Now, at fifty-seven young years, nothing has top the display yet. The feeling is way beyond fear to something indiscernible. It makes action movies appear as games played with toys.

The water around the sides of the ship moved away, as if to back off from its power. The U.S.S. Newport News and U.S.S. New Jersey continued to fire for twenty minutes. They were firing all guns at the same time. This is a salvo. I may not have known that word then, but I know it now.

I found out later that our objective was to take out a huge gun emplacement hidden within the mountain. Unbelievably, all of that shelling removed a mountain. There was nothing left except for dust.

We received a Navy, "Well Done, and a double medal presentation!" That is like saying we accomplished a Great Job! The Chief of Naval Operations (CNO), the highest Admiral in the Navy, gave this to us. The Admiral also, gave us the Presidential Unit Citation (twice), for our outstanding combatant duties. For us, that was payment enough!

Patrol Boats (IM)—Vietnam—Jan. 20, 2002

This is another unwanted memory. This may be a short memory on paper, but it is not short in my mind.

The sun was going down. The year was 1971. Orange and gray were the only colors that we saw. We were sitting on the canvas top of a patrol boat in the river. All the boats were lined up on one side of the outlet. The river usually ran a light brown, no ripples on the surface. Everything was deathly quiet. We waited for the setting sun. That night the river appeared to reflect the color of the setting sun. The shadow of the boats began to change into a ghastly gray.

There was no breeze that night it was extremely hot. We could see the steam rising from the land across the way. The piers began turning dark as the boats pulled away. They were going on assignments, as they did most every night. No one made a sound as we lie back on the canvas top. We listen until the distant engine sound slowly faded away. All of us were thinking about the same thing, "How many would return?"

Shooting Tracers (IM)—Vietnam—Jan. 27, 2002

I was stationed at a river outpost in 1972. There wasn't anything around for miles. The jungle was dense; it didn't allow let much light to get in. At night, it was very dark around the exterior of the camp. Everyone had to stand a four-hour guard watch; we would rotate and take turns. We had lights up on the towers, so we could see beyond the fence. It was the normal military setup, sandbags staked all over, machine gun emplacements, and all types of provisions stacked up to our necks. Our facility served as a staging area. We refueled helicopters and river patrol boat. We also had a repair facility adjacent to the river. One of the perimeter lines was just the river. We had to guard both the land and the river.

One of the hardest things a sailor or soldier has to do is waiting for what might be coming or what might happen next. When I was at a guard post, I never will forget, how all alone I felt as the night went on. The jungle was so silent except for the noise of the frogs singing. One tip, that someone is coming, is the frogs would get quite. Although it would be deathly, quiet I knew deep inside all hell was going to break loose. It could be a minute or even an hour. All I knew was when the firing started it was everyman for themselves. I would just go crazy. There was a rage response in me that I could not control. Something clicked inside me; I went on autopilot. All these things I experienced in training, so my responses were automatic. I didn't even have to think. It is very hard to explain exactly what happens during an attack. I only remember shooting at tracers coming in. Before I knew it, the attack would end.

I think there were more emotional and physical changes that went on during each attack. After each confrontation, there were changes that went though the mind. Everything I believed in went right out the window. The rage for survival took over and I felt like a trapped animal. I felt that I could have ripped their bodies apart with my bare hands. Only if I had their blood streaming down my chest, would I have been successful in stopping their attacks.

Floating Grass (IM)—Vietnam—Jan. 27, 2002

It was 1972. There always seemed to be balls of grass, which appeared as bumps, floating down the river. They don't seem like much to talk about, but this was a serious problem. Divers or swimmers would attach themselves to a large ball of grass to float down the river undetected. The swimmers would have explosive charges big enough to sink our repair barges or even a patrol boat.

As I was on duty, I would watch each clump of grass as it floated by. I would try to guess the course it would take and how close to the boat, it would come. The four-hours that I spent on watch were always a busy time. Watching the river, the jungle, grass balls, and the water around the boat, didn't give me much time to be afraid.

The one thing I remember well was one specific person. I thought I was hipper, until I saw him in action. All of us would be sleeping in our racks down below. Then we would wake up startled, look at each other as we shook our heads. All of us knew who was on duty; he never missed a trick. He would shoot at everything in site. He'd blast at the ripples here and shot at the ripples there. He shot into the jungle on the other side of the river. He threw percussion grenades at every grass ball that he saw. When the percussion grenades would go off, there would be a giant sonic boom. We could hear the boom echo along side the boat. The sides of the boat would rattle. We'd be shaken in our racks. Yep, we knew our friend was doing a great job, because we never got any sleep. When it was time to change the watch, one would always have to make a loud commotion; if you didn't, there was danger of being shot.

Almost Shot a Child (IM)—Vietnam—Feb. 11, 2002

The year was 1972. It was 4 AM in the morning in Saigon city. The streets were deserted, except for the South Vietnamese MP patrols. The curfew would not be lifted until around 6:30 AM. We knew we could relax a little bit, before the activity of the city began.

A Republic of South Korea Marine (ROK) and I were on guard duty that morning. We called them Rocks and they called us GI's. When the Rocks were on duty, I felt confident, because they were very well trained Marines.

We were guarding a hotel, which had about six or eight floors. This hotel housed American Service Men that had duty stations inside the capital city of South Vietnam. In the front of the hotel, there was a sidewalk twenty-five feet long. Around the front perimeter of the hotel was a black iron fence about twelve feet high. At approximately 10-foot intervals, all along the fence line, there were white concrete pillars. There were two concrete pillars directly in front of the entrance. There was one pillar on each side of the four-foot wide sidewalk. No South Vietnamese Civilians were allowed past the entrance. There was no gate across the entrance it was wide open. On the street side of the fence and on the pillars, hung signs written in Vietnamese saying, "DO NOT ENTER, MILITARY COMPOUND, HALT, and phrases to warn the public that this was a restricted area.

As the sun began to rise, so did the activity of the city. The traffic and noise was increasing on the street in front of the hotel. My fellow guardsman and I became more vigilant at our duties. Many Vietnamese women work at the hotel. We referred to them as momma-sons. We didn't use the words co or bon; these words meant Miss or Mrs. All personnel attempting to enter the compound must be checked for a valid identification. Everyone had a picture identification card displayed around his or her neck.

The next bit of activity would begin when the children set out for school. We knew the basic routine of the people.

We had just received a specific threat that morning. The officer told us to be on the look out for possible explosive charges concealed in backpacks. We were told these explosives could be carried by anyone. He told us do not be fooled and stay alert. He informed us about other bombs that were previously exploded around the city. The targets were bars, restaurants, and laundry shops that were frequented by U.S.A. service men. We were instructed that this hotel could be a likely target. We all took this very seriously.

The sun was up. The street was filled with a thick blue haze. All the people seem to travel on small motorbikes. They seem to be propelled by kerosene; it sure wasn't gasoline. Each of the motorbikes put out blue smoke, as if all of the bikes are burning oil. By this time in the morning, there was a strong smell of burning oil and the air stings the eyes.

The children can be seen going off to school in groups. As I looked down the street, I saw a very large crowd of children coming down our side of the street. I nodded to my Rock friend and he nodded back to me; we were both watching the same thing. I watched closely as the children passed in front of the entrance. I was thinking to myself, that things look orderly; we will get through this. Then as soon as I finished my thought, a little boy with a backpack on was standing at the entrance. The other children were still moving along. Why is he just standing there? I took my M16 off safety as I rose up my rifle. I'm running on automatic now. I hope he turns around! I thought that would be a good sign, if only he'd turn around! I glanced over at my Rock friend and he's raising his rifle too! Gosh, why don't you turn around! I started screaming in Vietnamese: "Yung Ly, Dee Dee Mow!!!" "Yung Ly, Dee Dee Mow!!!" "Yung Ly, Dee Dee Mow!!!" In English: "Halt, Run Away Fast!!!" While I was yelling, I slid my finger down and back; I felt the trigger. I was deciding when to fire; I glanced again with my eyes over at my friend. I could see we agreed. Since I had my rifle on the target, I would take him out!

The Vietnamese women that worked in the hotel began screaming down from the second and third floors balconies. The children out front were screaming for the little boy "to get out of there." "I knew enough Vietnamese to understand that some of the women were yelling to me, "Don't shoot him. Some of the women were just cursing me out. Other women were trying to tell the little boy, to go outside of the entrance."

I was in an extreme dilemma. Time literally stood still. I only had seconds to make my decision. I thought if he takes one-step forward, I would have to shoot him. I'd have no choice. I eased my finger pressure off the trigger, as I saw a Vietnamese woman come running out of the hotel. She put her arms around him and snatched him up like a toy. She continued running, carrying the boy, until she was outside the hotel entrance. I could hear her talking load to him. I guess she was scolding him.

My Rock friend and I looked at each other, both of us smiling and shaking our heads. I was thinking that sure was a close one. Both of us knew that the little boy didn't know how close he came to death. When we aimed our weapons down toward the ground, everyone started to cheer! I'm not sure what they were saying, but that was a big load off my chest.

Caskets Four High (IM)—Vietnam—Feb. 16, 2002

The year was 1971. This was my second tour in Vietnam. I had just finished survival training in Coronado, California. This was a very intensive training program. It was to teach us how to survive alone behind enemy lines. I won't bore you with the details, but we thought we had seen and done it all. We were, I thought, prepared for almost anything that we would encounter.

We traveled on a military chartered commercial jet. Our journey started in San Diego, California, and then we flew up to Seattle in Washington State. We stopped there for an hour or so, while the grounds crew refueled the plane. We were instructed that we could get off the plane, but we could not leave the airport terminal. All of us went to the restaurant lounge, where we had something to eat and drink. This was our last stop that we were allow to consume alcohol. We all had a few to celebrate our last stop in continental United States. We re-boarded the plane; our next stop was Anchorage, Alaska.

They changed the flight crew; no one thought that was strange. We learned after the plane took off, that these crewmembers were all volunteers. They received military combat pay for each flight in and out of Vietnam. This news spread like wildfire all through the passenger compartment. I don't know about anyone else, but the news raised my eyebrow. I thought, is it so dangerous to land at an airport in Vietnam? I didn't say a word. I kept my thoughts to myself.

From Alaska, we continued our flight over the Pacific Ocean to Yokosuka, Japan. I'm not sure why we stopped there; I thought maybe, we were picking up mail for the military stationed in Vietnam. We left Japan and headed for Vietnam. The whole trip from California to Vietnam took about sixteen hours. The route we took was called around the Pacific Rim. It was night; everyone was tired. We stretched back in our seats to catch a few winks. It was quiet and the lights were off. We were all sleeping peacefully, until the Captain began making announcements over the intercom.

By the sounds and activity in the cabin, we could tell that we were preparing to land. I looked out my window and I could see the plane was coming down. As we got closer to the ground, I saw that this place looked like the moon! There were dirt mounds and craters everywhere! I thought I heard someone say, "Welcome to Saigon, Vietnam." A military voice came over the intercom telling us, "The plane would not be on the ground long!" We looked at each other wondering what is going on. The voice continued, "Each of you will disembark from the plane in an orderly fashion. The luggage bays will be open. You will pickup one sea bag and proceed directly to the terminal. There will be two Military Police stationed at the main door. You will enter through that door and continue moving into the terminal. I say again, you will not stop at the door, you will move inside." This, I thought, was just more of the standard military talk. They never knew when to ask, Please. Sometimes I couldn't determine when they were trying to pull my leg. I heard the screech of the tires as they hit the tarmac. I felt the reversal of the engines pulling me back in the seat. I knew for sure, the eagle had landed.

There was a very serious atmosphere in the cabin. We all got up and moved tightly against each other to minimize the time for departure. We moved swiftly down the gantry, across to the baggage bay door. Grabbing a sea bag, we ran from the plane, about one hundred yards to the main terminal.

There was the sound of small arms fire pining across the runway! As I look to my left, I saw a frightening site. There were caskets draped with American Flags. They were stacked four high. Since I was running, I couldn't tell how far down the runway they were stacked, but it looked like many them to me! One would have been to many for me! I saw the same site when I left Vietnam in 1972. A person cannot forget a site like this. There are no words in the English language, which I can find to express the feelings I experienced!

The plane never turned its engines off. It seemed to me that as soon as the last person grabbed a sea bag and began running to the main terminal. That plane was moving very fast down the runway, quickly took off, and faded away in the sky. I was told that many of the commercial planes chartered by the military were slightly damaged delivering military personnel to Vietnam. I thought now, they tell me!

Visit To the Wall—Vietnam—Current Experience—Jan. 16, 2002

While I was writing this, I still have strong feeling inside. Maybe its frustration, anger, sadness, or maybe it's all three. All I know is my mind is racing as I write this in my journal. Dr. Wadeson asked me to, "Write down exactly what's going on inside my mind." Well here goes. I'm really shaking now, both inside and out. My pen won't even stay within the lines on the paper.

On December 27, 2001, I went to see the Vietnam Memorial. Everyone here in Washington, D.C. calls it, "The Wall." We live outside Washington in the state of Maryland. It wasn't a very long trip from our home. Dr. Wadeson asked me, "To see if I could get myself to go." He said, "Maybe it would bring closure to the things that I felt." He has asked me about the same thing for many years. I told him, "I just could not go!" I could not give him or myself a reason why. The immediate members of my family thought I might fall apart and worsen my condition. I even thought the same thing, but I didn't let them know. Let me run down the list of those that came with me that day. There was my wife, my daughter, and her husband. There was a niece, a nephew, and a sister to my wife. One very special person that came with me was our grandson. He was five years old and saw things for what they were. His mind was not cluttered with emotions.

As I walled down the sidewalk on the right was a slanted sign. It was there to explain the purpose of the memorial and a little bit, about what would be seen. I saw words like courage, bravery, fought, and died. The words all kind of ran together for me. I'm not sure why, but I didn't see quite clear. My grandson wanted to go with me as I approached "The Wall." His father held him back out of respect for me. He said grandpa need to go alone. I took note of this, but never said a word. Never were truer words spoken than, "I must go alone!"

As I was walking, I tried to get a grip and understand how I was feeling about seeing this great wall. I was thinking of the over 47,000 listed on tablets made of black stone. The wall was shaped like a giant chevron worn on a soldier's uniform. To me it looked like a great big black cliff. Many people fell off that cliff during those many years. As I walked, I looked at all of names carved in the stone. I felt like I could pass out dead away on the ground. I felt pain for the families that lost someone. Just as I was feeling sorrow, my grandson ran up and hit my leg. In a loud voice he came right out and said, "Grandpa, are those the names of all your soldiers that died in your war". After hearing that, all I could say to him was, "yes." He talked as though I was in charge. Right, me the general, I've heard it all now. I do not think I would have said anything, if my grandson weren't there with me to add his unique prospective. I thought long about what my grandson had said and I finally knew what he meant, "We were all there together!" That sounded very meaningful to me.

As I continued to walk, with my grandson at my side, I began to think of all the names not written here. What about the names of all the soldiers that came back? Some of these soldiers still suffer from the effects of that war today. I wonder if those in charge consider them in their body count.

Later at the Nurses Memorial, he asked me "What happened?" My grandson was pointing at the memorial. "Why is that man laying back, holding that thing on his chest?" I told him, "The nurses were helping him, because he had been shot."

As I backed away, from the Nurses Memorial, I overheard someone say, "Did you know that eight nurses died in Vietnam?" I thought to myself that only one had to die to cause sorrow. It was at that same moment, I saw a man on the park bench crying. I wore my hat with U.S. Navy Vietnam on the top. The man and I exchanged greetings just minutes before. I could not approach him, while he grieved on the bench. I knew how he was feeling, for I too had a deep sadness in my chest!

4

What Are Intrusive Narratives (In) or Thoughts?

THOUGHTS THAT FLOW THROUGH MY MIND (IN)—DEC. 30, 2001

There are times when thoughts, not pictures, run uncontrolled through my mind. They are just words that flow like a continuous river. They are called intrusive thoughts or narratives. These thoughts come all by themselves. I don't initiate or request them. These Intrusive Narratives (IN) or thoughts take control of my mind. I cannot stop them; they just seem to stop on their own. I do not know exactly which part of the brain these thoughts are coming from. I know the content of the thoughts are mine.

As I pier into the darkness of my mind, I hear a deep groaning coming from within. There are so many secrets hidden within my mind. Things I have never told to anyone. These thoughts are driving me crazy! Maybe, I can stop this continual pressure I feel from these flowing thoughts.

I ask myself, why am I plagued by memories of events I had no control over? Did I did do something wrong? Why do I feel so much sadness, sorrow, and pain? I know it is not some kind of judgment upon me. It must be something that has happened to me. Why had this happened? What was the purpose? I have learned that some people get a great deal of satisfaction from causing as much physical and mental pain as they can on other human beings. I guess this is an example of the old saying, "Mans inhumanity to man". This knowledge does not make the pain go away. These thoughts are of when I was a child, a young man, a solider, a husband, and a father. Now, I am an old man and still these thoughts overpower me. I know these things do not go away with time. Time itself does not heal, correct, or relieve the anguish that goes to the core of my being.

I have decided to reveal all of the secret oppressive thoughts locked up in my mind. I feel a need to put these thoughts down on paper. I want to find a place where I can leave them. Then maybe, I can find some peace from this continual torture going on in my mind and body. It is incredibly hard for me to write down all of these thoughts and experiences. It takes me months of concentration on a specific story, before I can even voice the events. Then, it takes many more months to work though the feelings, pain, and sorrow. Finally, relive the events in detail again so that I can write these stories down. It has taken me nine years to arrive at this point. The anguish I feel has helped me write this book.

I have a fear of writing personal things down. I feel like someone is going to use this against me to prove some point. This is paranoia. Dr. Wadeson has explained to me that it would be best, if I write down all of the things that are troubling me. I have to keep telling myself that this is the best solution for me.

THE FOLLOWING ARE THE ACTUAL NOTES FROM MY JOURNAL:

Dr. Wadeson asked me to put them in the book without any changes.

Jan. 31, 2002, I am writing this in a traumatic state. This probably won't go in the book—this really sounds insane.

I went to see Dr. Wadeson at 10 am this morning. I told him about a problem that is happening to me everyday. This doesn't happen all day long. This comes on in a random way. Let me think of a way to describe this. As I write, I'm going to think aloud, if you don't mind. This is definitely a rough draft.

Why is it, that I feel so pressured to write things down? I also have the opposite feeling; it's as if I'm filled with fear to write things down. I'm lying back in a comfortable chair. My golden retriever, Jessy, is at my side. She's bringing me dog toys to throw down the hall, so she can fetch them.

Well, back to the subject. I don't know if this is caused by something or if this is a feeling or a response. This event starts while I'm feeling ok—I'm not sure that I ever feel normal. I know that this is not correct English composition; maybe it can be thought of as shorthand. First I'm ok, Then I feel low, then happy, then sad almost to tears, then angry, then upset, then despair, and then I feel like I'm crashing down inside. Sometimes the feelings are so intense, I have to go and lie down for an hour or so. What is happening to me? I always seemed to handle things better when I know what I'm dealing with.

In the group session last week, one of the people said they understood what I meant. Although, it gives me the assurance, that someone else knows what I'm trying to explain, it also tells me I not crazy. It's just inside of my mind, I feel like I'm going out of my mind.

I always get a feeling of; how much more can I take? I really feel like I'm going to explode. I inquired of Dr. Wadeson if there was any medication that could help me. I ask if I should do something. He told me—write down what you feel. RIGHT! I thought. Here I am dying and he tells me to write. WRITE? This is what is going through my mind right now—When will this all stop—when will this end? How is writing going to help me? My body is completely tingling; my right hand is going numb. My fingers are shaking; these letters on my paper look deformed and wiggly. The letters look like worms. I can hear an echo in my head, as if sent from a great big horn. It says, "WRITE." Ok. I'm trying this; I'll give it my best shot. Gosh, I feel like crap.

This illness seems to take up all my time. It takes all my energy. Sometimes I feel like I can't go on. I have no idea, where my drive to go on comes from? I hope the drive I have doesn't stop. I wonder where Dr. Wadeson gets the strength to read all this junk.

Here is something that just came as an Intrusive Narrative (IN) into my mind. I just keep hoping that something I write down will hold some clue, which can point to a solution to this torment I'm going through!

TRAPPED HERE IN MY MIND

Having a mental illness, that seems to have no end,
Makes me forget about, how it was way back when.
This illness takes over my mind, strength, and will.
I guess my soul is ok, I know I have something inside.
What is it inside, that feels the sadness and the pain?
Is disillusionment and despair an emotion or is it felt?
What is the process of slowly losing your mind?
Is it control of the body taken over by the brain?
Is it a physical thing? Like chemicals out of balance?
I think going through this wouldn't seem so meaningless,
If something that I write down, could be helpful to someone else.
My life seems like an endless road of trauma, stress, and woes.

Peace and contentment are not part of the life I've known.

All of these kinds of things, like joy, excitement, and happiness,

Must surely be, only a state of mind?

What's the point of writing?

Does it give me pleasure, pain, or does it explain?

Well, if it helps me find a solution to this confusion

In my mind, it will have been worth it.

Until then, I'll stay here, trapped in my mind.

This is an example of exactly what we spoke about Dr. Wadeson. In one of the books I was reading, this phenomenon is referred to as an Intrusive Narrative (IN). The words just seem to come flowing out of the mind. I see this happening, but I don't know exactly what this is from or how to stop it. I really hope you can understand this, because as you can see I still need help. Is this normal; is it called inspiration, imagination, or static? I have never experienced this type of event in my life. I have nothing in my knowledge base to compare with this event. It may not be great at poetry, but it says what's in my mind. Maybe it's just so much static. I can't tell.

Sometimes, I really feel compelled to write. Maybe it's like a required hobby. At least with this hobby, I won't cut off my thumb. I'll have to watch out for paper cuts I know. I will try to be vigilant, as these stories flow.

Oh! Well, back to the problem at hand. I hope you can see how new thoughts, stories, worries, and the like totally take over my thinking—I'm just writing down my thoughts as they come. End of this journal entry.

◆　　　◆　　　◆

Many Intrusive Narratives (IN) At the Same Time—Jan. 23, 2002

Some days I'm bombarded by many presentations of Intrusive Narratives (IN) simultaneously. This would probably be all right if someone is talking to me, but these are in my mind. I'm not talking about a couple ideas or even just a few. There are so many ideas being presented all at the same time, they overwhelm my mind. I can't just turn it off or think of something new. At this point, my mind gets overwhelmed and I begin shaking inside. I feel a sense of overwhelming pressure that comes over me. My face feels hot or flushed; my palms get clammy and wet. Then, as soon as this experience started, it's gone again. It feels like I have just been hit with a baseball bat. I don't know when the event will return or leave again.

5

Are They Physical Or Mental Ailments?

Overtaken By Heat—Jan. 23, 2002

Sometimes my body gets physically very hot. The heat flows down my body from my head to my feet. I breakout in a cold sweat then, drops of water fall from my forehead and roll down on my face. My hair gets so wet; I can wring it out like a mop. It doesn't matter what the temperature is or if I'm inside or outside the house. This always goes on for a few hours. I have to sit down and rest. Sometimes this occurs at night when I have nightmares.

Overtaken By Weakness—Jan. 23, 2002

Another physical experience that happened sounds a bit like the experience with the heat. I will be feeling fine and have my normal strength. Then abruptly, I start getting weak. To me it feels like I'm famished and need something to eat. All the muscles in my body become very weak. I would compare this to being in the bright midday sun; when the temperature and humidity are above ninety-eight degrees. This weakness will stay with me for a few hours or sometimes the entire day. This comes on and departs, leaving me dumbfounded in its wake. When things like this happen, it's hard for me to trust my own mind. I'm left confused. I write these things down hoping someone has experienced similar things. Maybe someone has an answer to these very troubling events.

Stomach Aches—Jan. 20, 2002

The past four days my stomach has been rolling. I can hear an embarrassing gurgling sound. My insides are actually moving back and fourth. This is more than the normal shaking that happens all the time. I don't mean to be gross. I'm trying to tell it like it is. It has been four days of diarrhea. Today it changed to blood. This sequence of events has happened before. I've talked to medical physical doctors, they've checked for colon cancer and the like. As always, I do not have anything physically wrong. I sit there baffled saying, "What about the blood?" They tell me to keep an eye on it and let them know if this continues. I guess they know what they're talking about, because the bleeding always stops.

Physical Ailments

Even after coping with physical ailments for years, it's still hard to hear the Physical Doctors say, "This is a psychosomatic illness." This is a nice way of saying, "It's all in your head." I keep telling myself that my mind is causing these illnesses. I also talked to my physiatrist and he told me he understands how these things work. He cautioned me not to get upset. This is frustrating to me; I feel like I'm going to explode. I can't make my mind stop doing these things; I didn't know my mind was doing anything? It would be nice if I could get a brain transplant. I'm always looking for new ideas. There must be an answer to overcome these problems. I keep hoping. I'm learning to cope with these physical and physiological problems caused by what they call Post Traumatic Stress Disorder (PTSD).

There are specific physical ailments that will be encountered. To cope with each problem explain the ailment to both your physical doctor and your physiatrist. I have found the bleeding a lot from the stool. Is a PTSD problem, but it also can be a sign of colon cancer, or other ailment so check with both doctors? The worst thing you can do is think it's all in your head and ignore the problem. This is how you build your coping skills, by first talking to your physiatrist and he will direct you to have it looked at by a physical doctor. Do not follow the recommendations of friends or family only someone trained to work with PTSD will be able to give you the correct answer.

Only So Much Trauma One Can Take

I try to get a prospective of what is really going on in our lives. Sometimes I get so confused I don't know which end is up. I keep telling myself, that I'm a normal educated person. I have always seen myself as taking things in stride. I try to go with the flow. I know the world is not a perfect place. I don't expect any kind of special treatment. I've pulled my own weight, so to speak. My wife and I have always worked. We made a good living for our daughter and ourselves. I keep asking myself, what went so wrong. How could this have happened? Dr. Wadeson says, "We didn't do anything wrong!" It's hard for me to think about the thirty-two years we've worked putting a family together; we wanted to make a difference in the place where we lived. Then the PTSD bomb was dropped! We are still picking up the pieces now that the dust has cleared. We lost our boat, truck, car, house, all of our savings, and retirement. Then, if that wasn't enough, we went bankrupt. We use a positive outlook; we say everything is up from here.

Dr. Wadeson impressed strongly upon me that there is only a specific amount of; stress, presser, and trauma that a person can handle. One example is a cup can only holds a specified amount of water after that the water overflow the cup.

What I heard through the grapevine is the nervous system can only take so much BS. I feel like I could blow my top!

Confusion—Only One Thing at a Time

At present, I can only think of a single assignment or task. I try to do things around the house, but sometimes I get confused. Let me give you an example of confused. I carry a load of laundry from the upstairs to the basement. Once in the basement, I have no idea of why I'm there. I have to sit down for a while and then the knowledge comes back to me. I get up, put the laundry in the washer, and get that going. Then, I check the dryer. If there are cloths left in the dryer, then I have a new problem. I did not put the cloths in there. Where did the cloths in the dryer come from and where do they go? I have to sit down again and figure this out. This process is not automatic for me anymore it is manual.

Well, I think you see the problem. Everything that is accomplished around the house or out in the yard requires many steps to complete the task. Going to a real job, in an office or in construction, is actually a joke. I really do not have the ability to stop this confusion in my mind. I get confused at home, in the grocery store, or almost anywhere. The confusion does not occur on any specific schedule. The confusion comes and goes.

Maybe you can see how hard this problem can become. Believe me there are many more. The best thing I can hope to accomplish is learn how to cope with each situation one at a time.

Explosions on the Skin

A medical doctor performed a biopsy of the bumps that keep appearing on my skin. These bumps can be found all over my body. After the results of the tests came back, the doctor said the bumps were nerve endings. Some of these nerve endings grow into hard scaly bumps. I showed my son-in-law a few bumps that were on my arm. His response was definitely medical. He just said, "Gross." I knew he could see the problem. Some bumps explode under my skin. These appear as popped blood blisters. While others explode on the top of my skin, which causes the blood to stream along the surface of my face, arms, and legs. I try to cope with this by using a prescription cream. This cream is so strong I only use it at night. The cream knocks me out and I go to sleep.

Uncontrollable Shaking

My body shakes both inside and the outside. It's a kind of tremor. I appear to others that I'm terrified of something. I can't seem to control the shaking, mentally or physically. I spill the coffee from not only my own cup, but also I spill the whole pot of coffee, while I'm pouring a cup. Peas fly right off my fork. I do much better with a spoon. I can even keep a beat with my knife, to some rhythm only my mind knows about. Eating at our house is quite an event. It seems to bring back memories of raising our daughter. When I brush my teeth, I have an automatic brush. Shaving is a little bit trickier. I hold one hand with the other; this stops some of the motion. I made a slight improvement in this process. I still use two hands, but now I use a long mirror on the wall, and prop my one arm against the mirror. Sometimes I am cut up pretty good. It's a good thing I have a beard or I might not even be writing this story.

Forgetting or Losing My Place

Sometimes I forget things when I moving from one room to another. I know everyone has experienced this at sometime. "Someone said if you go back to last location you were, the thought will come back to you." I know this idea worked before I had PTSD. I've tried using this trick now. With PTSD, this doesn't work the same anymore. Sometimes I'm trying to find out what state in the USA I'm presently located. You might think of these coping skills, with an attitude or else you will go nuts!

The feelings and questions experiences are what are happening? What's going on? I feel very strange for a while. It's as if I've lost my bearings. I feel completely lost. I don't have a clue about anything at all. What I have noticed is with PTSD, when I forget, the information might not come back to my mind until tomorrow. That is, if it comes back at all.

Let's say, that tomorrow I'm doing a completely different task. The information I was trying to remember yesterday comes rushing in on my mind today. Now, I get upset, because I can't figure out where this stuff is coming from.

Dr. Wadeson has explained that these are called intrusive thoughts. These are uninvited thoughts that come into the mind. Just imagine the feelings I get when I loose all kinds of information. Stuff like, things I did, people I knew, or even places I've gone. Sometimes I lose it in the middle of a conversation. I can't for the life of me, remember even the subject of the conversation. This is very embarrassing. No, I'll tell you, it makes me feel extremely stupid.

Not able to hold onto a thought long enough to complete the task I'm doing is a problem. A real scary one is, when I go some place in the car and cannot remember why I'm there. It's understandable that I don't travel by myself very much.

One nice trick or coping skill my wife thought of is presetting my cell phone to our home number and I have the cell phone with me wherever I go. That way if I become disoriented I can just press one button and she can tell me what to do or where to go!

Feeling Out Of Place—Jan. 22, 2002

I haven't typed up any stories for a few days. I still have a problem putting my feelings down in words. My mind tells me no one really cares about these intrusive memories (IM) anyway. I feel like I'm backed into a corner. I keep feeling like I'm going to be taken away, because I do not fit into somebody else's mold of how a normal person should act. I just want to be myself. That is a big problem when I'm not sure of myself. I really feel that I do not belong here. I'm not speaking of a specific place. I mean I do not feel that I fit in this world. My wife has heard me say this for many years. We always joke about it. I say I have my ticket. She replies that she will let me know when she sees the bus.

I read in a book that one of the Dissociate Disorder (DD) symptoms is, feeling out of place or feeling one does not fit in. It doesn't help me to know this. I still do not know what to do to correct the problem.

People seem to have all kinds of activities that they do. It's almost impossible for me to break away from all of the activities that are going on in my brain. I have trouble understanding why these intrusive memories seem to have the upper hand. They take control of my mind whenever they want. This is very complicated to explain and even harder to understand. I'll be sure to do many activities when I get control of my brain back. Normal people cannot see to grasp the concept of what Intrusive Memories (IM) are all about? To show you another coping skill, I go to a man's PTSD therapy group each week. When I explain a problem or situation I'm going through all five of them can give me a suggested solution that they use to cope with the problem. Additionally, Dr. Wadeson provides many solutions to try. Moreover, each PTSD person in the group understands exactly what I talking about! That gives me another level of assurance that I not loosing my mind. My wife goes to Dr. Wadeson to learn how to deal or understand me. My wife and I don't discuss PTSD at all. Now, loved ones are wonderful, but they too have a limit of the amount of stress they can manage. I know much more about PTSD than she does. PTSD scares her and she worries about what is going to happen next or happen to us! Instead of trying to get my wife to deal with the disease, we let Dr. Wadeson do his job and we just learn to work together. This makes everyone's participation and frustration level much easier to handle!

I love it when people, well meaning I am sure, tell me to, "Get over it." How about, "Stop thinking about it." That is as easy as stopping a train with your hand. How about this one, "Just let it go." These memories are always in complete control of my brain. This is like cancer of the liver; the cancer has complete control of the liver. A person can't just wave a wand and the cancer is gone. Another good one is, "This will all go away," or "Time heals all wounds." One of my personal favorites is, "Pray about it and you will be set free." Talking to friends is great. I've learned to be very selective of whom I'm talking with. Mostly I talk about these things to Dr. Wadeson, write in my journal, or the best one is talk about in our group.

Let me see if I can use a little logic. If a person has inoperable cancer, would you tell him, "Get over it?" On the other hand, if a person has diabetes, would you say, "Time heals all wounds." I don't think so!

It appears to me that many people who look at a mental illness as something, a person should be able to overcome or prevent. Can a person with diabetes overcome it? Without the medicine they would die! Mental illness is not like brushing you teeth and you won't get cavities!

Mental illness is just like any other chronic disease. Mental illness is a disease in the brain. The brain is just like all other organs, when diseased it doesn't perform exactly as it should. When the proper solution is found for any disease, properly applied, and then we will have a cure. Until then, people need to learn to understand causes of mental illness. It is not a mentally ill person's fault that they contracted the disease. It is not something they have done. Fate is favorable to some and not to others. That is the way life is. A little knowledge goes along way to restore balanced thinking. In all of my reading, I've found there is not very much sympathy for the mentally ill in this country.

I just tell myself there is a lack of understanding going on in this town. I just kindly listen to them, nod, and say, "Sure." I've been in this condition for over nine years. Even I do not know what to expect next from PTSD. I think I'm pretty close to the source of this illness. I have written down everything I know about this illness know at PTSD. This is a tough nut to crack. (Pardon the pun.)

I go in to see my physiatrist, Dr. Wadeson, each week. He says I'm getting better, in terms of having clearer thinking (at times). I'm able to be more logical and concise in my thinking. My wife can testify that many times, I'm totally lost. Here's another one, "Get a grip." It's hard for any family to deal with a permanent disease. The most truthful solution I have found to date; is learning to cope with this each and everyday. Group therapy is one of the strongest tools that you have to work with. Normal people in society cannot possibly help you. That is as ridiculous as relying on a sixth grader to obtain the proper job for you. Those that have PTSD can help you understand and cope with it. Even your family members, as well meaning as they maybe, do not have the answers, for which you are searching. Don't waste you time, join a group therapy session for PTSD! It will change you life.

Mood Swings—Jan. 31, 2002

"The thing I was talking about—maybe—referred to as a type of mood swing. This is not PMS. I was just ok. Now, I feel like my head will explode. I feel angry and upset; my stomach is shaking in and out. I can physically feel this happening. My arms and hands are shaking. I feel like I could reach up and rip my head in half to let the presser out. I feel like my whole being is going to explode. What the HHH, is going on? I'm angry, hurt, disappointed, amazed, confused, crying, shaking, and my heart is pounding. I take deep breaths. I don't think it helps. I really wish we could do something about this, besides just writing this down. I am in real anguish. I feel like I am staked down to the ground and someone is beating me with a cat of nine tails. The whip digs into my skin just enough to cause bleeding and pain, but not enough to kill me. This stuff just keeps going on. I know this sounds insane. I do not think I can take anymore."

After Dr. Wadeson read this, he altered my medication in Mar. 2002. These violent mood swings are now been controlled by medication. I feel much better as of Mar. 31, 2002.

Lack of Trust—In People—Feb. 1, 2002

I've been writing now since Dec. 2001. I've tried to give a priority or importance to this task. Maybe in my own way I think I can write myself out of this situation. Maybe I'm just dreaming. It's 3:15 A.M. I got up, because I have another terrific headache. Really, I bet it's, because I need some coffee and cigarettes. I know—don't say it. I thought while I'm up I would write what's on my mind and think. This is almost like having a front row seat into another persons mind. I hope this helps you.

I never seem to have just BS type of conversations. What I mean is, just having a best friend to talk with. Someone that will listens and understands. Someone I could get advice from or just to talk with about simple things. Yes, I have this kind of a relationship with my wife, but I don't think it's the same thing. See I have to tell you the truth, I don't exactly understand why I should nee such a relationship. Dr. Wadeson has explained that this is only normal. Oh, really, I don't place confidence in any person. Let me tell you why.

I remember specifically trying to have confidence in people. I tried to have confidence in a friend from the office. We knew each other for at least ten years. I thought after ten years, I should know the person. It was not the case. I talked to this person freely about a wide range of conversations.

After a time, I started overhearing stories. I would walk into an office space and the room would get deathly quite. I never thought about being paranoid. I really don't care what people think about me. I was amazed! The stories were about me. The stories were the things that I had said, I thought, in confidence. I was very upset, but I never said anything again. I just stopped talking about myself. I decided to be strictly business in the office. I never have understood why some people take personal information and turn it into public office trash.

Lack of Trust—In Organizations

I went to a public hospital to discuss some deeply troubling issues, which were weighting heavily on my mind. For the very first time, I went to speak to a mental health professional. As I talked to a doctor, she took down notes. That is a common thing to do. By the time I walked from the doctor's office in the hospital, I overheard nurses talking about my troubling story. What made it worse; they were giggling and laughing at how such a thing could happen. When I thought this could not become more embarrassing, one of the nurses pointed me out to her friends. They are looking right at me, I thought. I was so embarrassed, I never went back for the help I needed. I've carried this problem with me all these years.

I maybe getting on a soapbox, but I have to say what's on my mind. Gossip always hurts someone. If the other person wanted these stories made public, they would have told everyone. When people make light of someone else's traumatic story, his or her story becomes a carnival event. No more does the story have its original anguish the person felt. Why do people seem to have no feelings for another's torment? Is it because they do not want to tell their own stories? I, as others, believe that life has purpose and meaning. Take care with the things you know. I hope in recording these words, the eyes that read them will look to the kinder side of life.

Lack of Trust—In Primary Caregivers—Feb. 26, 2002

Now, it has been explained to me that I don't have trust in people, because of the things my parents did to me as a child. Thinking and practicing cannot put trust back where it has been broken. These are the thoughts I have when thinking about trust.

The Qualities of Trust

Trust is not something one is required to give to another.

Trust is something that is proven by the passage of time.

Trust is not something that can be stolen by a thief.

Trust is not something that can be bought or sold.

Trust is earned by consistent actions.

Trust is something that should be expected and held in high esteem.

Trust is something that should be prized above other merits.

Trust is something that should be held close to the heart.

Trust is something that can be lost,
>   It can be breached,
>   It can be denied, refused, or taken away.

Trust can be used to miss the mark, as in mistrust or misguided.

Trust can be missing from a relationship and it will soon dissolve.

Trust can be non-existent, as in distrust.

Trust is needed, as well as, required to maintain balance.

Trust is something that one can be sworn to uphold.

When trust is broken, misguided, or disregarded the relationship between the two parties becomes imbalanced. When the scale of balance is tilted, a greater weight is applied, in favor of one side.

Personal, family, parental, or public trusts are equal, in as much as, they require an extremely high level of integrity and respect for the persons holding such a position. This level of responsibility requires that all parties be obligated to demonstrate that the trust is above reproach.

A party that breaches the trust of their responsibilities is normally removed from the position and appropriate punitive actions, if warranted would be applied. Parents in this case, have been given the responsibilities of the primary caregivers, family trust, and the parental trust. Law, from society, requires parents to provide a normal level of security, medical attention, food, clothing, and shelter. These things are not luxuries that can be negotiated. These are the most basic needs for a human being to survive. When the children are hungry, it doesn't take a college professor or a degree to have enough common decency to feed them. Children require direction and motivation to maintain a proper prospective for success. Children never have to be beaten unmercifully into submission, in order to guide them on an honorable path of life.

As primary caregivers, they passed this responsibility to me when I was nine years old. This was not a onetime babysitting job; this job was all day, everyday. The parents passed to me, a responsibility greater than my years or experience. I didn't have a hotline; I could call and get information, instructions, or advice. I had to wing it, all by myself. I had no knowledge or experience raising children, in the proper way. I felt, that I was always under too much anxiety, trauma, and responsibility; I was overwhelmed by the experience. Parenting is the act of raising children by their parents. It is not an act of children raising children. I also, think this was inexcusable and irresponsible for my parents to subject me to these severe conditions and demand perfect results.

The family trust can also be referred to as, the family values. These are moral and ethical principles traditionally upheld and transmitted within a family, as honesty, loyalty, industry, and faith.

The loyalty is built by the continual mutual respect between all members of the family. There are two types of faithful allegiance created by the bonding of the family. The first is a faithfulness of allegiance that is created between the children; the second is a faithfulness of allegiance developed between the children and the parents. A profound tenderness called love is a naturally occurring feeling within a family.

The manner, in which, the parents conduct themselves is an exhibition of honest intentions, actions, or principals.

The parental trust, parents are given this responsibility, because they have caused another human being to be born into this world. This duty comes with many great rewards and just as many ominous downfalls. This was not a plight, which came upon the parents when they were unaware. A rock did not just fall out of the sky and behold the parents now have a child. Parenthood is a job and a responsibility one chooses to take voluntarily. No parent is forced to have children, but once the children come from the union of the parents, they are now responsible for all facets of raising a child to adulthood. This is why parents are given such high respect from society. Society knows the enormity of the task that lye's ahead of them. The difficult decisions that will have to be made are the responsibility of the parents. A great amount of physical labor will be required of the parents over many years. The parents have the responsibility of a child's life in their hands to mold them into a responsible adult. They must create and motivate the child to learn important attributes such as understanding, standards, honesty, kindness, humanity, faith, hope, love, and even trust.

Children must not to be used as pawns by the parents, to obtain a warped sense of enjoyment in sadistic rituals that cause pain and suffering.

A Contorted Fit—Feb. 7, 2002

Last night a very strange thing happened to me. Nothing like this has every happened before. I don't know what this is called, but I'll explain it the best I can.

With my wife by my side, I was lying in bed on my back. I had my eyes closed. I was listening to the soft music my wife was playing on a headset. I was relaxing, petting my golden retriever Jessy. I looked at the clock by the bed; we were resting there for about an hour. She put her head set away. I was kissing and hugging my wife good night, and much to my surprise. My whole body began jumping, as she said, "What's going on? I told her that I wasn't doing anything. This is happening all by itself."

My legs were jerking, that's when I realized I was not just shaking how I had experienced before. All the muscles in my arms, legs, feet, stomach, neck, head, and back were all jerking in different direction. I was scared. I told her I had no idea what was going on. I'm completely without words to describe the terror I felt.

Observe the process I thought, I have to explain this to Dr. Wadeson. I felt a great concern to ensure I explained this right. I was able to talk, but I didn't have control of my body. I tried to stop my body from moving, but I could not.

This contorted fit lasted around two minutes. I really was not looking at the clock. My wife looked at me and said, "You're shaking the whole bed." Even Jessy sat up, at the end of the bed, gazing at me with great concern. I apologized to my wife and told her that I was extremely embarrassed. She assured me not to worry and that everything was ok. I shook inside and out for another three minutes.

I lay on my side for another hour, starring at the wall and the clock. I needed to know what had happened. I was extremely concerned. What should I do if it happens again? What should I do if the symptoms get worse? What signs do I look for? What should I do if it occurred without warning? What does this tell me? I thought this was similar to an epileptic fit I saw once on TV.

On Feb. 9, 2002, Dr. Wadeson gave me a prescription to try for thirty days. The results look good and I'm taking this medication now on a regular basis. The contorted fits or secures didn't happen again until July 2002. I have only had two secure reoccurrences.

Yelling Out In Stores—Feb. 27, 2002

During the year of 2001, my wife and I went to the grocery store to do a little shopping. I was still trying to adapt to large crowds of people. She would give me a verbal list of a couple of items each time we entered an aisle. I was simply to go down the aisle and pickup the items. This probably sounds like a very simple task, which even a child could perform. Since I have PTSD, this little task becomes a very complex one. Let me explain.

In my mind, I always have intrusive memories interrupting my normal process of thinking. These memory interruptions cannot be stopped. When shopping, my wife is asking me to add two more memory items in my mind. Now I have to try to concentrate on both remembering what the items are and searching for the items as I proceed down the aisle. I struggle as hard as I possibly can to do this easy task of shopping. Halfway down the aisle, I forget the name of the item for which I am searching. Then in a flash, I remember the items name. With great frustration, I have forgotten again and have to ask my wife, "What am I looking for?" That's when she gets upset and says, "You were not listening again." I'm upset hearing this repeatedly, so I say to myself, "That right, I don't even know what store I'm in. You're lucky I still know the state we are in." I keep my cool; I don't want to upset the apple cart. I softly, with control, ask her if she could tell me the name of the items again. I'm also thinking to myself, "This store has like seventeen aisle of food! This is going to really be fun!" Now a logical way to solve this problem is for me to write the names of the items down and simply retrieve them. (Dr. Wadeson recommended that I should write the items down on a list. He also said I should let my mind rest as much as possible. (I have not learned what rest your mind means.) That would defeat the purpose, which is to try to override what is occurring in my mind and control my memory to accomplish an immediate task I want to complete.

Now, the whole time we are shopping, I know my wife is fully aware of the memory interruptions I have going on continually in my mind. She appears to be concentrating completely on doing her shopping. I understand that this is a normal thing to do. She acts as if she is unaware of any problem I have and she expects me to act normally. The frustration builds inside of me, until I feel like crying. I say nothing; I just gut it up and go on.

I feel helpless and completely overwhelmed by the fact that no one is aware that anything is happening inside my mind. This is the part of PTSD, which makes the barer feel so alone and out of place. This is what makes me feel like I'm living in a different world than everyone else. All kinds of the things happen to me each day, which I have to keep to myself. I cannot discuss these things with anyone, because they cannot understand. Anyone I tell these kinds of things to, thinks I'm crazy; then they act very differently towards me from that time forward. Rightfully so, I have PTSD and I'm still trying to understand all that is happening to me. I usually wait until my next appointment with Dr. Wadeson. This is probably the most important reason why I maintain a very detailed journal, which I share with Dr. Wadeson on a weekly basic. Well, let me get back to the story.

See this shopping experience isn't over yet, we've only gotten two items so far; we've got a lot more items to pickup. Retrieving products continues for thirty or so minutes. Once we are finished, we are ready to proceed to the checkout line.

At the checkout line, all of the people have their carts full of groceries and waiting to pay. Most normal people would say, so what is the problem? People are always waiting in long lines in a grocery store, right. Well, let me tell you what I, with PTSD, experiences and feel.

I have already begun to shake. I usually take charge of the shopping cart; that gives me something to steady my arms. All of the people are talking in their little groups. All of the groups are discussing different subjects. There are about ten checkout lines in the store. I can hear the constant beeping of the register scanners.

All of this noise and information being sent to my mind overwhelms me and I begin to stare. This is when I go into a trance. My wife knows when I'm in a trance and said to me, "You're staring again." I try to break loose, but my mind has control. I can't think anymore. I lean over to my wife and say, "WHY ARE ALL OF THESE PEOPLE TALKING SO LOUD?" Everyone, in all of the ten checkout lines, stopped talking! Not a word was spoken. The only sound that could be heard was the beeping of scanners. My sense of hearing had become so hypersensitive; that I could actually hear each of the conversations. It was as if everyone was talking right in my ear.

Everyone was looking as us. My wife was extremely embarrassed to say the least. She asked me, "Did you know you were screaming, when you were just talking?" I told her, I thought I was just speaking to her. Everyone stayed quiet for a very long time.

Once we arrived at the register, I pulled out my electronic bankcard. While I was standing there, I knew exactly how to use my card. Then it was time to use my card. I totally lost the knowledge of what I was supposed to do with the bankcard. I felt like all eyes were on me; I was so embarrassed, I just looked back at them and casually smiled. My wife again came to my rescue. She gently removed the card from my hand and performed the scanning and numeric entry. The man at the register was gracious and said; "All this new electronic stuff is pretty complicated for many us. It's O.K." I felt like a total jerk by this time, so I just nodded my head and smiled.

Again, as I have said before, recounting these incidences through writing them in my journal, I actually relive each moment in time. All the noise causes me to shake violently. I get a cold chill that runs the length of my body. The hair on my head actually stands up. I have a great pain in the pit of my stomach. I must stop writing for a while.

Mental Comprehension—Feb. 27, 2002

Let me clarify my inadequacy of being able to comprehend speedy conversations. I'm not bragging, but I have about fifteen years of schooling and I am fifty-three years old. I'm just stating this so that it's understood; I didn't just get off the banana boat yesterday. Knowing that, I'd like to give details about the dilemma I undergo when people talk too rapidly. I'm not referring to the way a valley girl talks, in a brisk fashion. I'm referring to the conversations of normal everyday people. I'm not able to capture a long stream of words into my mind and comprehend the conversation before the individual stops talking.

I stand before them dumbfounded, as if they hadn't said a word. I heard them talking. I just missed all of the words they said. I would describe it as hearing about every third word. It's like trying to respond to half a sentence. I knew each word as it entered my mind, but the problem appears to be when the meaning of the word is being searched for in my mind, my memory forgets the word. I end up with a meaning of a word, only I don't remember the word that the meaning goes with.

My brother-in-law is one of those people that can remember enormously long stories and jokes. When he gets going, everyone is laughing and admiring all of the subtleties of the story and things like plays on words. Everyone around the table just looks at me, with a wondering eye. I know their trying to determine if I comprehended the joke or story. Most of the time I don't get it, but they are gracious and don't say anything. I just nod my head to acknowledge, that I was listening to the story.

I've been working on responding to telephone answering systems, which ask a million questions and then have me respond by pressing a number. It goes on and on with an endless array of questions. I always have to wait until they ask for, "rotary dial, or speak to a person." Those are always my choices; because my mind cannot give me the answers fast enough to respond within the allotted time. I know everyone just loves these answering systems. I do get confused when they throw in one of those, "I did not receive a response, please press 9 to hear the menu again." Why would I want to hear it again, if I didn't get it the first time?

Startled Easily—Mar. 4, 2002

When the phone rings, I'm startled. I fumble and get it on the next ring. I have trouble understanding the information displayed on the caller-id, while I'm figuring out what to do next. Who is calling? What should I say? All of this information is running through my mind. Finally, on the third ring I answer the phone. I try to talk, but my mouth won't work. I'm having trouble talking and the person on the other end has already begun to talk. Now, I have to figure out what they're talking about—now I'm frozen in a trance. Then, to complicate matters, my wife is telling me, "Answer the phone!" "Say something!" "Who is it?" By now, I am overwhelmed by information. I begin to get frustrated, thinking to myself, "Why do I even try answering the phone?" Sometimes it gets even more complicated such as, when I've waited until the fourth ring and the answer machine picks up the same time I do. Woo, I won't even try to explain that sequence of events; it's beyond frustrating!

Another example of being startled is when the doorbell rings. I'm so startled that I forget what to do next. I know, open the door, but I go through the same processes in my mind that I have listed above.

My last illustration is when someone comes up from behind and startles me while I'm doing yard or other types of work. Last summer, I was trimming the edge of the grass with a power trimmer. I was just working along listening to the hum of the engine. When my wife walked up behind me and called out my name rather loudly, because of the engine noise. When she called out my name, I was so startled; I threw the trimmer about five feet into the air. I think it can be seen that in the daily work environment, this would be extremely disruptive or possibly dangerous. Imagine tools flying off, into the air, from the second story of a building under construction. How about possibly coffee, donuts, and office supplies becoming projectiles as they fly across the office partitions. This is probably one of the reasons, why many of us that suffer from these conditions, are not currently in the workforce. Workers' comp would probably have a sharp increase in premium rates.

Anatomy Feeling Numb—Mar. 5, 2002

Since May 10, 1995, I have felt numb at many different levels, in many different parts of my anatomy. In the first two years after I became ill, the numbing was quite severe. During the first year, I couldn't feel the presents of my body in anyway. All I could sense is that my mind, body, and spirit were three distinct entities. This baffled both the physical neurologist and my physiatrist; they could not determine any corrective actions to be taken. This caused me an enormous amount of concern! I didn't know if I was dying or if I was going crazy. The doctors gave me their most professional assurances that nothing physically or physiologically was wrong. They said this development might resolve itself over time.

I was frantic, but I followed the doctor's instructions. My personal feeling was; I cannot sense my physical body at all, but I'm supposed to remain calm? I didn't know how to respond to this diagnosis! When the best of the best told me, they didn't know what to do; I felt extremely alone inside! I had to mentally, work through many emotions of the unknown by myself. I was both terrified and completely distressed! Both my wife and I were amazed! My wife has stood by my side for almost thirty-years. My wife and I will continue to go through many unknown adventures together.

I will describe a few of the experiences that happened. Now keep in mind I could see my body and my mind knew mentally that all of my body was present. I could control my upper body all the time. From time to time, I would lose control of my body from my hips to my feet. This would cause me to fall down on the ground. The one thing I notice when I fell down, it would be like a slow motion controlled fall. I didn't just fall and hit the ground. Although I never got hurt falling down, this was still a very serious matter. Let me explain.

One day I was sitting on a riding lawn mower. I tried to put the mower in reverse, but somehow I couldn't determine if I was moving forward or moving in reverse. I had no sense of motion. At that same time, I lost control of the lower half of my body. Since I didn't have control or feeling of my legs, I could not stop the riding mower. My wife and I had just discussed the dangers of proceeding up a steep hill. I assured her I was not planning to go up the hill. I was trying to avoid proceeding up the ten-foot incline, but I went up that direction anyway. When I reached to summit, the riding mower began sliding sideways down the hill. I fell off the mower as it flipped over and began rolling down the hill. I did have the opportunity to view the mower blade actively spinning. While sliding down the hill, I didn't have any positive or negative emotions. I felt as though I was watching someone else falling down the hill in slow motion. The riding mower broke apart as it traveled down the hill and crashed on the sidewalk below. It was a miracle that I wasn't killed!

I think it can be seen that the loss of motor skills and sensory perception can be very hazardous. Dr. Wadeson put me on riding mower restriction after he heard the news.

I began to wear half-gloves almost all the time to protect my hands. Another surprise came when my brother-in-law and I were putting asphalt shingles on a roof. We were busily lining up and nailing shingles on. We were moving along with great efficiency. We were just talking about how we would have this roof done before dark. When, the efficient roofing process we had going, suddenly stopped. We looked at each other with great amazement! I had just nailed my finger to a shingle on the roof! I didn't even feel it! I pulled the nail out of the roof with my hammer and twisted the roofing nail left and right, to remove it from my finger. Blood shot out across the roof. He asked if it hurt and I said no, I couldn't feel anything. He went on talking about how gross, it was and how he could not believe his eyes. As he expounded about his disbelief, I wrapped my finger with duck tape to stop the bleeding. We joked about how duck tape could be used to fix anything. We continued working and completed the roofing project.

After this situation, Dr. Wadeson just shook his head and told me to be more careful.

I don't mean to make light of this situation. I was entering my third year of this illness. I have to laugh or else I'd cry. This is one of the techniques; I used to cope with each new situation. During these years, those around me saw many unbelievable things happen!

Let me tell you a couple more stories, I think you'll see that they are also unbelievable.

During the same summer, I was in our basement workshop cutting some patterns out of wood with a table scroll saw. Again, in this situation I had no feeling in my arms or hands. I was just trying to move forward with my life, ignoring all handicaps I had and not give up. The saw had become red hot from cutting all the curves in the wood. I brought the saw around a corner cut and didn't watch the location of my fingers. The saw cut into my thumb almost to the bone. There was no blood at all from the cut. I recognized the problem and slowly backed the saw up through the same entry point. The blade was so hot, that it seared the cut closed as I backed the saw out of my thumb.

Dr. Wadeson checked over my thumb to ensure that I was not injured and then he put me on power tool restriction. He was still shaking his head over that story, when I left his office.

I was very careful about being visually aware of the location of all my extremities. Then that winter, I was helping my wife jump-start a vehicle. I was wearing a work jump suit and half-gloves to keep warm. My wife awaited my signal that the cables were connected. I gave her the signal. After a few tries, the dead battery was charged enough to start the vehicle. She gave me the signal to remove the battery cables. I removed the cables from the vehicle with the troubled battery, so that it could charge on its own. In the mean time, my wife and I lit up a smoke and waited for the battery to charge.

We were busy smoking and talking. I forgot to disconnect the cables from the fully charged battery. My wife said to me, "Your smok'in!" I thought she meant I was extremely cool. Then she yelled, "You're on fire!" I knew this was not a complement. I looked down at my hands and they were on fire! The jumper cables had melted my gloves and the insulation on the cables! There was smoke rising up through my sleeves and coming out from the neck of my jump suit! I quickly disconnected the jumper cables and threw them on the ground. I began stomping out the fire on the jumper cables, while trying to remove my gloves, which were in flames. One of our neighbors came running over when he heard all the commotion and saw the flames. He shut off the running vehicle. Once all of the fire was out, we all noticed that there was no insulation on any of the cable connectors. My neighbor looked at my wife and me, in utter disbelief. I had held the cables together, while the other end was still connected to the twelve-volt battery. I didn't feel any electrical shock. I didn't feel the fire from the gloves that were on my hands. We were all amazed, that I was not injured in anyway! This was another unsolved mystery.

This time Dr. Wadeson checked over my hands to ensure that no plastic materials were embedded in my skin. He also was amazed that I was not injured. I don't think he knew what type of restriction to put me on after that incident. He said that I was very lucky and that I should try to be even more careful. When I left Dr. W's office, he was shaking his head over this story too.

ANATOMY FEELINGS OF: TINGLING, SHAKING, AND NUMBNESS—MAR. 5, 2002

I think that the shaking, tingling, and numbness are all connected to the same problem source. I'm not a doctor, but I see all of these things happen to me. I believe I have eight years of real life experience to draw upon. These things all have to do with motor and sensory control nerves. If the nerves don't communicate to the brain correct information, the brain cannot control the body movements properly. When the brain doesn't receive accurate sensory (feeling) information, it cannot determine something as simple as, is the water flowing over my hands hot or cold.

I would like to describe the feeling of numbness that I have experienced for all these years. I think everyone has crossed their legs and found that the leg goes to sleep. Numbness is more intense, than having a part of the body fall asleep. I believe that having the dentist inject Novocain in the nerves of my mouth is closer to numbness. Novocain will deaden the pain, but it doesn't remove the feeling or sense of pressure. The intensity of numbness is like using, both Novocain and removing the sense of pressure simultaneously. Now, I think you understand that this part of the body feels as if it does not exist.

The frightening part about numbness is that the body part that is numb, doesn't feel like it's attached to the body at all. Let's use the right leg for an example of how to cope with numbness. What I do is, physically view the right leg with my eyes. I touch the right leg with my hand. This reassures my mind (brain) that the leg is physically present. Remember the numbness may go away tomorrow. Who knows? The important point to understand in your mind is that the leg has not been cut off or injured in anyway. With this knowledge in your mind, you can begin to understand and cope with numbness. Make sure that your mind understands the way things are. Don't expend any of your energy thinking about what might have been. If the numbness goes away, you'll be the first to know. Until that time comes, you must use a coping skill to reduce the trauma that your mind is going through. This will also reduce the fear of the unknown, which causes undo stress. Numbness, once you work through it, is not something to fear. For you, it is a known fact. You cannot stop the numbness by thinking or worrying about the matter. This numbness is caused by emotions that cause a chemical imbalance to occur in you brain. Let your doctor fix the chemical imbalance, while you work on coping skills. Each coping skill you use, will allow you to take control over the emotional aspects of your life. Regaining control of your life will return the peace of mind you are seeking. Work with the senses you have to compensate for the deficiencies you have, which in this case is numbness. It's not so bad, after you change your way of thinking about numbness. This new way of thinking will become automatic after working on this coping skill for a while.

Tingling can be an intense or moderate feeling. It can be localized in one area or it may encompass multiple areas simultaneously. Additionally, tingling can encompass the whole body at one time. I have also experienced a kind of rolling mobile tingling. When this rolling tingling occurs to me, the tingling may begin by rolling slowly down the top of my head, continue down the back of my neck, move along both of my arms, and stop at my hands. As this rolling tingling is happening, I sometimes lose control of the part of the body that is affected. I have had both days and weeks, in which the tingling is continuous. Although this can be extremely emotionally upsetting, the same rule applies, which is trying to control you own emotional response. The more the tingling occurs, instead of getting upset, which you know does not solve the problem. Begin to train your self to be alert and ready so that you can immediately begin to control your emotional response. I can tell you the tingling will not kill or hurt you. Try to remove all of the fear you may have about the experience. Once you have removed the fear, begin to work towards controlling the movement of the body part, while the tingling is occurring. I know from experience that it is possible to regain control of your body.

Now, for the issue of shaking—I have not found any type of solution to this problem. I cope with shaking by keeping a detailed journal and collecting all the information, I can obtain. I have not seen or read any beneficial knowledge on the subject of shaking. There is a specific section in this book explaining my own personal shaking situations.

Shutting Down—Mar. 5, 2002

After I have been awake for about six to eight hours, both my mind and body shutdown. I would describe this experience as reaching the maximum point of emotional tolerance. This is also described as the point at which one becomes overwhelmed.

If we think of the brain as a computer; then any type of input that totally saturates the maximum capacity of the computers ability to process information will cause a system failure. The result is that the computer will shutdown or crash.

The brain can also become saturated by any combination of these types of events; such as; emotional, physical, sensory, activity, sound, talking, arguing, yelling, screaming, music, TV, radio, dogs barking, kids playing, abuse, stress, trauma, reading, studying, worry, overwork, work pressures, or lack of rest. This is by no means an exhaustive list. These are just to be used as an example of what can make a person shutdown. There is no such thing as a "Nervous Breakdown." Nervous breakdown is a misnomer. There are many types of shutdowns the doctor must define yours. Everything that shuts a person down has to do with the nervous system, but they are not all the same.

Let use my experience on May 10, 1995, as an example of a total and complete mental shutdown. I'd like to show the events that took place in my life, as a mathematical equation. I think you'll see what I mean. We will add up all of the major events that contributed to my shutdown.

Child Abuse + Trauma + Stress + Combat Exposure + Night School + Overwork for 27 yrs. + Work Pressure + Over Studying = Complete & Total Mental Shutdown

Now, many of the events that occurred in my life didn't happen by choice. Matter of fact, I don't think I could have avoided any of the events. I always used every ounce of energy that I could muster to perform up to my best in whatever challenge came my way. I had a boss that would remind me, when he saw frustration or discouragement in my actions. He would laugh and say, "It's not a problem; it's just another opportunity to excel!" In other words, he was telling me to continue and press forward toward an attainable goal. I did as I was told, much to my detriment!

It can be seen that with the drive to succeed, there also must be personal limits set on the appropriate distance to travel, before you must rest. The ability to rest is not a negotiable aspect of your life; it is required. If I had rested more, my brain would not have shutdown. Once the mind shutdown occurs, it is not quickly repaired. Extreme patience is required to bring about your own recovery. One of my very first questions that I asked Dr. Wadeson was, "When would I be well enough to return to work?" I'm still awaiting the answer to that question. Remember that this recovery is now nine years of hard work.

Excess Sleeping—Mar. 11, 2002

Most normal people think, that sleeping in until 10 am a couple days a week, would represent excess sleeping. That's not excess sleep any longer. When I first became ill, I slept most of the time for six months. My brain was so overloaded, that it would not work until it received an appropriate amount of rest.

When I tried to start doing some lawn work to make some money, my brain would shutdown about every four hours. I had to find a way to prepare myself before each shutdown occurred. To ensure that my body was ready for the shutdown and that I would not be injured; I attached a small electronic alarm clock to my belt. I set the alarm to activate every four hours. Everyone would be alerted to the fact that I was going to shutdown, when everyone heard the alarm. Sometimes, I would just tumble to the ground and fall asleep. My partners would, make sure that I wasn't going to fall off a roof while cleaning leaves out of a gutter. They would simply drag me, like a rag doll into the shade, because they knew that I was not injured and in a couple of hours, I would be back to work. Most of the time, I was able to make it to the truck and sleep on the front seat. At first, I thought I had narcolepsy. That's when a person's body falls asleep, whenever it finds it necessary. Dr. Wadeson assured me that I didn't have narcolepsy.

Nothing has changed much over the years. I have tried to keep busy and sleep whenever I feel the need to relax. The big difference now is that, I just feel sleepy not exhausted, as in the previous years. Dr. Wadeson has also explained to me in many different ways, that I must observe and be aware of the needs of my own body. Then, I must respond to the need. For many years, I had been trained to push on to the next level, ignoring what the body needs, just use my mind to press forward. If you listen to the way I was acting before; it sounds more like a military type of thinking. That's fine, but it will not work forever. Your body will crash at some point. The crash point is different for each person.

I sleep and wake all hours of the day and night. This is when I have the time to write in my journal. I think that documenting the progression of PTSD has become a hobby of mine. My body is on its own time schedule. The changes from Daylight Saving Time to Eastern Standard Time don't seem to affect by body clock. Maybe, I'm on PTSD time. My getting up and falling asleep all hours of the day and night drives my wife crazy.

I cannot go on long day or overnight trips. The more activities involving a physical expenditure of energy tire me out to the point of exhaustion. I try to participate in physical events, but it seems that my mind quickly becomes overwhelmed and I must lye down and sleep for about an hour. Once I become energized again, I am able to attempt additional activities.

Motivation—Mar. 12, 2002

A lot of the time, I have absolutely no motivation to do anything. I don't have any hobbies or pursuits, which I actively pursue. The one hobby I am just learning is writing. I do enjoy writing. Writing this book has helped me express many things that have troubled me for many years. With all of the intrusive memories going on in my mind continually, my mind doesn't have the ability to prompt me to perform any additional tasks. I feel that inside of my mind, I am very busy. I guess motivation is the act of being driven, pushed, or having the desire to accomplish something. I think that my mind has been pushed too far for too long. I don't know how to control motivation.

Uncontrollable Rage Caused by Injustice—Mar. 19, 2002

From 1977-1995, I traveled all over the U.S. on a moments notice, went to school both day and night, worked both day and night via dialup and internet connections installed at my home, and my work responsibilities never really stopped. I was upset and despondent, but I always chalked it up to having an important job came with additional responsibilities. I surely was not going to give up, quit, complain, or shirk my responsibilities according to the contract. It always had the phrase; "the incumbent shall provide all required service within four hours." I saw that statement, but I didn't think it would always be my turn. I thought I just had to reach down deeper inside myself to give all I had. When I had a nervous system, shutdown on May 10, 1995, I knew I had given my all. I had no more to give.

On June 16, 1995, I made a call to the New York Headquarters, from Dr. W's office, to give them an updated status on my health. They said, "that I did an excellent job, but because I had no more leave, I was fired!" I could not believe what I was hearing. I gave the phone to Dr. Wadeson in hopes that he could understand what was taking place. After Dr. Wadeson talked to them, he returned the phone to me and said I had heard correctly. The President of the New York office said I would be receiving a letter of verification in the mail and hung up the phone.

For the last nine years now, my family has paid the price for my mistake in judgment. I lost my job, and then my wife had to retire early from her job to take care of me. To make ends meet, we had to use all of our saving and 401k retirement funds. We sold our boat, truck, and car to try to stay afloat. We had no more funds, so finally we had to sell our house. Remember, I was making close to $70,000 and my wife was making $30,000 a year. I had a long-term disability insurance plan to take care of any major medical problems. When we submitted our claim, we found out that the insurance didn't cover any type of mental breakdown. I paid a lot of money into this plan, but I did not get an acceptable return on my money. Long-term disability insurance is not exactly what it advertised to be, so watch out!

I was quite angry to say the least. I sank into a deep depression on top of everything else that was happening. My memory of the first four to six months is hazy. I have to rely completely on my journal entries, to reconstruct what happened. Inside of me disbelief, disappointment, extreme sadness, disillusionment, frustration, and anger turned into a full-blown rage. During this time, Dr. Wadeson was doing his very best to provide both physiological and medical assistance in the form of proper medications. The rage inside of just kept growing. The rage and a fight or flight response was slowly taking over my whole being. I began to be taken over and completely controlled by my former military combat training elements and responses. I began to wear a marine hat similar to the one I wore while in Vietnam. No one in my family said anything. I'm sure my wife could see the change that was coming over me.

I began having detailed dreams, of how I would go about resolving these issues, concerning this company's lack of sensitivity to my situation. They expected to blow us off and due to my medical status; they thought they didn't have anything to cause them additional worry. They never thought about the tenacity of my wife. For months, my wife made many phone calls to both the New York and Austin, Texas offices. She had a conference call with the President of the company and all of the corporate leaders about the health compensation issue. They relented and I began to receive compensation for my illness. After six months of receiving compensation from the insurance company, my former employer called us to inform my wife that we had to pay back immediately a total of $16,000.00. There was no way we could, in our wildest dreams, of paying that amount of money back! My wife told them to stop all the payments, because we didn't have any money to pay that amount back. We didn't hear from them again.

I was once again enraged to a point that I was not sure how to contain myself! I discussed this problem with Dr. Wadeson and again he assisted me in controlling myself for a while. I began having dreams again, about what actions I should take. I felt that a grave injustice was being committed; and that no one was able to help us correct the problem. I could see that no matter how much of myself I placed into a job, the bottom line for company's stops with there financial interest. Right and wrong has no place in the business world, so they did nothing. I felt I should take matters into my own hands, but what could a single worker do. One of the dreams began to have prominence in my on going nightmare selection.

The Solution To Injustice—My Dream—Mar. 19, 2002

In the dream, I would get on a plane and fly from Maryland to New York. The man I wanted to see worked on the 28th floor of certain building in New York. I would get a hotel room near by and prepare my solution to the problem. It was winter, so I would wear a black business trench coat, shirt, and tie. I would remember to carry my brief case. That way, I would look just like everyone else. I would be able to travel freely through the building. I could see myself enter the building, through the very large glass doors, in the front and conveniently rise in the elevator to the 28th floor. When I got off the elevator, I would casually show my company badge to the person at the desk. I would make sure to nod my head and graciously say what a good morning it was. I would turn left and walk down a long hall to the big office at the end. Once there, I would open the door, walk in, and shut the door behind me. I would walk up to the very large desk and ask the man his name. Once I knew he was the man I was looking for, I would tell him who I was. I would wait for this to sink in. He would probably stammer and stutter saying, "Oh, yes." Then, I would open my coat to reveal to him the solution to our mutual problem. He would say, "What…What…Are you going to do with that?" At the hotel, I had prepared a little surprise for him. I took a baseball bat and drove nine spikes into the end of the bat, so that the spikes pointed in all directions. Not knowing what to say next, he just sat there, as I swung the bat as hard and fast as I could. The spikes imbedded themselves into the side of his head and blood would spurt everywhere, like a shower nozzle. I walked around the desk to get a good look at him. Then, holding on to the bat, I rolled his chair swiftly across the room and through the glass window of the 28th floor. I just left New York and came home. I WAS NEVER CAUGHT OF COURSE, BECAUSE THIS IS JUST A DREAM!

Dr. Wadeson realized the depth of my rage and asked me to do a few things to try to get the rage out of me. I was to use my physical strength to ravage, impale, destroy, and mutilate something that was not a human. While using my physical strength, I was to think about the object of my rage. I would be directing my attention on the person in New York that fired me. I told him I would do my best.

Uncontrollable Rage at a Vehicle Dealership—Mar. 19, 2002

It was very cold that winter; we had an accumulation of around two feet of snow. Since our bankruptcy, we had been trying in everyway possible to rebuild our credit. We decided that one way for us to earn better credit would be to purchase a vehicle. We did all of the normal things, like starting in the show room, look at the outside lot, and finally choose the vehicle we wanted. I received a monthly payment quote from the salesperson of $200.00 and he assured me that there would be no problem. Then, all of a sudden, the vehicle went up in price.

A little frustrated, I asked if they had something else that would meet our budget requirements. He assured me that there was one and he would have it brought around for us to see it. We had been in this show room about an hour. He has the vehicle brought up. We like it. He assured me the payment was our budgeted about. My wife and I took it for a test drive. Everything seemed ok; we talked about it and decided to purchase the vehicle. The salesperson said that's great and he takes us to the finance department.

Now, this man tries to add on undercoating, bed liner, extended warranties for engine, body, tires, and the list never stopped. At this point, we had been at the dealership for over two hours. My patience seemed to be warring very thin. We kept saying we just wanted to buy the pickup, as it is, and nothing else. Then, he calculates the price and tells me the cost will be about a hundred dollars over the amount I had agreed on with the salesperson. That's it; I got up and reached over the table for his neck! I was going to choke him to death with his own financial tie! I told him the deal I made with the salesperson. I went into an uncontrollable rage! I told him to get the salesperson in here, NOW! Yes, I was yelling at the top of my lungs! I wasn't going to have one more slick fool screw me around or run me in circles! I wanted some straight talk, or someone was going to remember I was here! In came the salesperson, he had hear everything I said. I think the whole building heard. The salesperson was talking fast now; he said right off the bat, that the boss had told him our amount was $200.00 or no deal. Immediately the finance man left the room. I assume to get an ok from the boss. I was still standing; my wife was trying to get me to calm down. I couldn't help myself. I had completely lost it! If that finance person came back with bad news, all hell was going to break lose! Mr. Finance returned very shaky. He said he would run the numbers for us. I love when they say they'll, "run the numbers." I thought numbers my aaaas! I patiently waited for his reply. Now he says, "let me check something else." He was busily typing and although it was winter, he was sweating. He looked at us and said slowly, "$218.00 is about as close as I can get." "Would that be ok?" We said, "Sure that's fine. Now, please help us to get out of here." He said, "We are rolling on it now." His computer was spitting out all kinds of papers to be signed and within fifteen minutes, we were out of there. I really believe he was very glad to see me leave.

Uncontrollable Rage with a Punching Bag—Mar. 20, 2002

A few weeks later, a rage came over me that made me feel like I could kill someone. I followed Dr. Wadeson instructions, because I knew in my heart that I didn't want to hurt any specific person. I found an inanimate object in the basement, a punching ball. Although it was winter, I was sweating so much that the sweat was just running down my face and my shirt was soaked. I had not performed any physical exertion yet. In the basement, I put on a pair of punching gloves and began to hit the punching ball with ever-increasing fury. I continued to punch that ball with all of my strength. The ball was attached to a board on the ceiling by a steel grommet. I didn't think anything about how secure the ball might be attached. I continued to hit that ball for about a half and hour. My rage had not subsided one bit. I was beginning to wonder if this was the way to release my anger. All of a sudden, the ball broke loose from the ceiling and shot across the room. I thought the steel connection must be defective to have broken that easily.

We also had a punching bag hanging from the floor joists in the basement ceiling. I thought surely, this would not break. The bag was attached to the floor joists by a large linked chain. I began to punch the bag with all of my might. I got into it and was thinking of the person that fired me from New York. As I continued to beat the living heck out of the bag, to my surprise the chain broke and the bag flew across the room and crashed against the wall. I didn't know what to think. I went upstairs and explained to my wife what had happened. She didn't know what to think; she didn't say much about it. I guess for that day, I was able to release some of my frustrations.

Uncontrollable Rage Removed a Garage—Mar. 20, 2002

During the winter, we received two foot of snow. The snow was so heavy that the roof of the boat garage caved in. We never get snow that is two foot deep. We filed a report with the insurance company and they said that they had received many claims from our area. They said once the current garage was removed the new one could be built. The insurance company sent us a check in the mail.

When the weather warmed a little and the snow melted, my wife and I went out to work on taking down the garage. The garage was fifteen foot tall; twelve foot wide, and twenty-one foot long. It was constructed of four-inch PVC pipe and the walls were made of corrugated fiberglass panels. The structure had been standing for about two years.

The first day went along very well and we were pleased with our progress. The second day I was in a rage again. I told my wife that I was going to take my frustrations out on the garage. With my bear hands, I began to punch the four by eight fiberglass panels. She kept telling me to be careful; and I kept on punching. The panels were flying throw the air with the greatest of ease. It must have been quite a site, because one of our neighbors came over and asked my wife if everything was ok. I really started getting into it and within an hour or so; all of the panels were lying on the ground. The only thing that was left was the PVC pipe structure. I continued to think of the person from New York that fired me. With my bear hands, I punched the four-inch PVC pipes about every four-foot. All of the sections were crashing to the ground with a thud. I kept on punching until the last piece of the structure was on the ground. This didn't take me more than an hour. My hands were bleeding, but I could not even feel anything from my arms to my hands. By now, I had calmed down. We spent the rest of the day stacking all of the materials in separate neat piles. When we finished, our neighbor that worked in construction told us he could hall all the material away immediately. We agreed. My wife was concerned that I might have been injured, but I told her I felt better.

Uncontrollable Rage Dismember Crates—Mar. 20, 2002

A friend and I decided to work on a project to build and sell some Adirondack chairs. We wanted to reduce our up front cash cost, because we didn't have any money. He told me of a company, about five miles down the road, which had the perfect solution for our project. This company packed and shipped household good for the military all over the world. He told me that, the just dispose of all the old shipping crates. He thought we could get the company to give the old packing crates to us and we would remove them. We approached the manager and told him of our proposal. Much to my surprise, the manager said take all we wanted.

It was still winter, so it still was cold outside. The following day we came prepared to obtain a few shipping crates at a time. The crates measured twelve foot high, six foot by eight foot wide. My friend and I started to dismantle a shipping crate together and all of a sudden, I went into a rage. I began thinking of that man in New York that fired me. I went out of control. I was ripping, tearing, busting, and slashing all over these crates with a crowbar. My friend just backed up a few feet and he stopped taking apart crates, since I was doing such a great job. He began filling up our trailer with the wood that was flying from my direction. Before I stopped, I had dismantled twelve crates in less than an hour. My friend yelled to me that I had to stop; the trailer was full! I looked at him in amazement! Even though it was winter, all of my cloths were soaked from sweat. I thought to myself, everything seems to have happened so quickly. I wasn't even tired. I felt much better, after releasing my anger. We came back a couple of times to pickup wood, but the work never went as quickly, as the first time.

6

Gradual Recovery Is Possible!

What I Have Done To Gradually Recover—Mar. 25, 2002

I'm sure you noticed that I said, "Gradual Recovery," recovery will not be accomplished overnight. No one has come up with a quick fix to repair problems with the brain. The brain is one of the most sophisticated organs in the body. It has many automatic safeguards to protect itself from injury. Once you understand how complex the problems with the mind can be, the sooner you can settle down and begin to use your endurance for the long journey ahead. I'm not saying the situation is hopeless. I am living proof that PTSD can be managed, coped with, tolerated, endured, and the condition can be improved. There is no cure. Everyone's situation will vary. Work with your doctor and concentrate on the process of gradual recovery. Don't give up and don't quit! Also, notice I did not say that recovery was easy.

Finding a Psychiatrist I could completely put my trust in was my first objective. We chose Dr. Wadeson, because he had many high recommendations from the people we knew. If recovery is the goal you are seeking, you must choose a doctor, in which, you can put your life in his hands. The doctor you chose is going to reshape your mind so that you can recover. This is a daunting task.

Keep a Journal—Mar. 25, 2002

Dr. Wadeson asked me to keep a very detailed journal for the first two months, after I became ill. He asked me to try to make an entry every fifteen minutes. This was done so he could track important information about each of the many medications I was taking. I kept track of the name of the medication, the time I took it, the amount I took, how I felt before, and after I took the medication. What reactions were noted, any improvements felt, my feeling. I was not successful in accomplishing housework. The work was too hard, complicated, and confusing for me at that time.

I became more depressed, despondent, and cried as I watch myself unable to perform simple tasks. Inside of my head, I knew how to do these things. I did not have the ability to communicate to my brain and make it do what I wanted it to. The big problem was figuring out how to explain this to Dr. Wadeson. I was extremely frustrated! When "I cried out for help," I found that I was in another world. The world everyone else was in was just floating on by without me. I couldn't get anyone around me to understand the dilemma I had. I was completely horrified, as I found myself trapped behind a glass wall. I could see everyone else, I could hear the sounds, but no one could understand or hear me! Since I was able to type on the keyboard, I began to type into my journal everything I was feeling and thinking. Dr. Wadeson altered the medications I was taking using the information I typed.

I use this coping skill. I could type information from the thinking center of my brain, but I could not write by hand or vocalize the things that were happening in my brain. That was a surprise to me at first, but then I realized that one part of my brain was doing the typing and another part did the talking and the writing by hand. Even to this day, I have problems with writing and spelling by hand, but typing and spelling, as you can see, is working just fine. Your goal is to find out what is still active in your brain and what is still being protected from harm by your brain. The brain will not let you use the part of the brain that is working on. Advice you're Psychiatrist and he may have a medication to solve some of the problems. It is unrealistic to think all problems with PTSD can be corrected. You have to use the abilities you have and proceed with care!

I thought like you that I was damaged for the rest of my life! Remember, that this problem (PTSD) was cause by emotions, stress, trauma, etc. There is no physical injury. There has been an emotional overload. Emotional scares take time to heal and it takes more time than healing a wound like a cut or gunshot. It will not be, until we know more about the way the brain functions, before corrective actions can be applied. The source of the trauma or emotional overload must be stopped from reoccurring. Or else it will be similar to continually removing the scab from a cut; the cut will not heal.

Cutting Lawns—Mar. 26, 2002

I was in a deep depression for many months. About a year had passed and I still could not speak very well, so I spoke in short sentences. Everyone I spoke to gave me a funny look, so I knew people could tell that something was wrong. This was very painful, but I knew they didn't understand, because even I was trying to understand what was happening to me. I tried to ignore them and push ahead. Not being able to talk was very hard for me personally, because I used to stand up before corporate board meetings and make promotional presentation about computer software systems. At this time, I could not talk my way out of a wet paper bag.

Around 1997, I made a suggestion to Dr. Wadeson asking him if I could drive again, to get out of the house. I didn't feel free. I told him I felt like I was restricted to the basement, the same as when I was a child. Two years had passed since I first became ill. He thought that this need to get out, and be on my own could be a positive sign, that I was making progress. He knew I still had problems communicating with the muscles in my legs. He told me to be especially aware of my ability to control my legs and if there were any signs of problem, I was to pull off to the side of the road. Then, I was not to drive until I talked to him. That seemed fair to me.

When I started to drive again, I felt like when I was a teenager, my whole body was tingling with excitement. I drove around for a couple weeks and everything seemed to be working all right. I suggested to Dr. Wadeson that maybe I was ready for a challenge. He took a long look at me and asked me what I had in mind? I told him, I would like to try cutting lawns for the elderly. He asked me where, when, how, who, and all of the third degree stuff. I felt like I was on a job interview. He was actually trying to determine how my thinking processes were working. I passed the test! Dr. Wadeson said I could try one yard, in my own neighbor hood. I already knew the elderly woman, across the street that I was going to contact.

I contacted the elderly woman and got the job. She had about an acre of grass to be cut. There was a small amount of grass around the house and most of the lawn was in a big section in the back. I cut her grass every two weeks. I started cutting the lawn cautiously, but after a few times I built up my confidence. When I was in the backyard, I began to drive the riding mower ever faster with each pass. I was checking everything out and making sure, I could feel my legs.

I already had a few accidents with my hands. Things like nailing my hand to a roof and running a drill through my finger. I had no feeling in my arms or hands. At this time, I wore leather gloves to protect my hands all the time. I would work about three hours and then I would become so overwhelmed that I would fall asleep. When I was cutting lawns, I felt free, as if I were riding on a go-kart. My wife told me that I drove to fast, but I didn't think so. Come to find out later, after crashing on the riding mower, I discovered that I was not able to determine or sense the feeling of forward or reverse motion. What I had been using to determine speed was the wind against my face. I was using the highest speed on the mower, sixth gear.

I slowly progressed over the next year, where I was cutting lawns for about seven elderly customers. I still had a problem with becoming so overwhelmed that I had to crawl up in my truck and go to sleep, in between cutting lawns. I had problems with controlling my legs. I'd be walking along carrying a bag of grass seeds and I would fall flat on my face. I would just look around to see if anyone noticed, then I pushed on past the problem and continued doing my work. I was trying to make the best of a bad situation. I didn't want to give up. I thought, I knew what I was doing and things were going all right. I was surprised another problem arose that I hadn't thought about. I was purchasing the equipment I needed to complete the lawns. I didn't have the concept in my mind, that I spent more money than I was taking in. I caused a serious cash flow problem, because I was over extended.

After a near fatal crash on the riding mower, my lawn cutting days were over. Dr. Wadeson and my wife told me to find another line of work that would not kill me. I sank into another deep depression for many months.

What I've Learned—Mar. 27, 2002

I am trying to show that the person with PTSD has to learn what senses are working correctly. I have learned that there are many concepts for me that do not work such as; the passing of time, speed, motion, I've loaned out money to people who never intended to pay me back, being financially overextended, allowing people using me, or people ripping me off. These are just a few of the concept the PTSD person thinks are still working, when in fact they are not working at all. I've told Dr. Wadeson many times that I cannot always believe what my own mind is telling me! This is an overwhelming realization that normal everyday concepts have been reduced to the level of a naive child. It takes many time, concentration, and effort on my part to use the senses I know I have that work, to compensate for the senses that are deadened. Deadened senses do not provide proper responses or information to the brain. The problem comes in when my brain is not always aware that anything is wrong with the information it is receiving from the remote nerves. Example: Is the hand hurt? No answer also means the hand is not hurt. The real fact could be that the hand is cut off and not present at all. This is the dilemma. Even today, my wife says that my actions are slow. My verbal and motor actions are about three seconds slow. I don't react or respond immediately to real time events. An example would be the dogs start fighting, or a bowl of water crashes on the kitchen floor. In my mind, I don't know exactly what course of action to take. I am busy observing the circumstances and collecting information about the situation. That's when my wife brushes me aside and says "Don't you see what is happening?" or "Don't you care about what is going on, someone could get hurt?" The thing that hurts my feelings is; I really do care, but my brain has not found a solution to the problem yet. From my point of view, I'm still waiting on my brain to help me. This is very frustrating, but I know people don't understand what is happening to me inside my brain. I guess this problem can be thought of as slow or no response to real time problems.

This is one of the hardest problems; it hurts deeply to view what I'm doing. I feel as though I'm watching my own precious child falling down the steps and not being able to act to save him. I think of myself as a kind and caring person, but because of what is going on inside of my brain, I may appear as lazy, heartless, unkind, or uncaring to others. This is very sad for me to see happening and I can't change anything to make it better. Again, I feel locked up inside; I can't do or say what I want. I am a prisoner in my own body!

I have been working on these problems for many years and I am making progress. I don't have everything working correctly yet, but I have to remember that there are many pathways in the brain. It takes a long time to work out the problems. There is not one solution for everyone. The point I'm trying to make is I have found a way to work with or compensate for these problems, so can you! It's just like learning to walk again after an accident. It takes patience, work, and a will to succeed! Part of the daily frustration I feel is, because I know everything in my mind use to work and now I have to start over! It's ok to be outraged, frustrated, and disappointed! Just don't give up and don't quit trying!

Correspondence Courses—Mar. 27, 2002

I enrolled to take a correspondence course for small engine repair. I was thinking that this would be a much safer type of work for me to do. When the first five lessons came in the mail, I was excited. Maybe this would really be fun. I read over the first and second books. I thought I'm ready to take the chapter test. While reading over the chapter test, I found that I didn't remember anything at all about the chapter. I went over chapter two and found I knew absolutely nothing that was in the book. I thought I would just read the chapters again. After reading chapter one, I could not remember anything. I was upset and frustrated, I knew how to read, but nothing was sinking in. I had fifteen years of school and I know I was able to remember stuff back then. I thought I would have to talk to Dr. Wadeson about this problem.

I went into see Dr. Wadeson, I told him my dilemma, and he wasn't surprised. He already knew I had a memory problem. He had told me before, but I didn't remember it. The thing he said was a surprise to me, I only recently understood! He explained the situation to me and as usual, and I took notes. That's when I noticed I always took notes, because I could not remember what he says. Dr. Wadeson told me that my current memory and my ability to comprehend information are still not working! He said these things would come back by themselves. I thought, "Yea, and the next ice age is coming too!" Each time I think I am getting somewhere, something else comes up and knocks me off my feet. I was very frustrated! I asked him, "How long will this memory problem go on?" He said, "It's different for each person, no one knows for sure." As the years go by, I keep wondering how much more can I stand? I felt like I'm going to explode. After talking to Dr. Wadeson, I sank into another deep depression for many months.

It has taken my years to understand the things he told me, but it does not have to be that way for you. The following paragraph is for the reader! "This is very important to understand many abilities have been shutdown, not damaged they're just in hibernation. They are not broken they are only turned off. Your brain has not been damaged such as by oxygen deprivation, sections are asleep! Once the distress level has been lowered to a tolerable level, these abilities can be reactivated. You must try to control your reactions to detrimental revelations, many deactivated potions of the brain, or abilities you seem to have lost will come back in their own time. You are not brain damaged in anyway! PTSD is not like a brain injury in a car accident. Now, keep in mind this coming from a person that has watch a large number of abilities come back when I least expected it. You must be calm, and relax. I can hear you yelling Relax! Relaxing will allow events to transpire in your brain more quickly. Work on the reasons and sources of the stresses in your mind that caused PTSD to be activated. I am not saying all is going to be wonderful; you will only get what you work on. Some functionality may remain deactivates for a very long time or permanently. It all depends on the severity of PTSD. Again, consult with your medical professional they are the only ones that can walk you down this path. My suggestion is to listen to mood or stress relaxing CD and use the techniques explain in a book about relaxing or mediation. Recovery does not occur overnight. It will be a gradual recovery, be prepared for the long haul. Now we know about relaxing the mind."

I talked to my wife and gave her the news. She said she would like to complete the course. She did, and got an "A." Then, she completed a course in two and four stroke engines. Now, she is our own engine and motorcycle repairperson. She loves working on engines now.

Woodcrafts—Mar. 27, 2002

I decided to start making woodcrafts. I ordered plans for different projects. Then I started buying accessories for crafts such as; clocks, phones, temperature gauges. Then I bought a shed and decked it out with lights and all kinds of sparkles. I didn't see anything wrong with trying to have a little craft business. The big problem was I did not have the mental capabilities to read the plans to build the projects. I tried as hard as I could to build things, but I could not understand how to do things by the step. Even with the directions in front of me. Since I had no feelings in my hands, I cut half way through my thumb with a scroll saw. In fact, I was not able to complete even one project. I was devastated! My wife helped me by getting rid of all the supplies. Again, I overextended myself by spending more money than I made. I was not mentally capable of planning or completing any of these projects. I again went into a deep depression for about a year.

Warehouse Work—Mar. 27, 2002

I thought I would try working at a charitable organizations warehouse. The boss wanted me to drive a sixteen-foot truck and deliver goods to the thrift stores. I told him to let me work in the warehouse and see how that goes. I knew driving big trucks would be a dangerous problem. He didn't know that I was the kind of person that crashes while driving around on a riding mower. I began to work in the warehouse. After four to five hours, I felt completely wore out. It was summer and very hot, I passed out twice inside the back of the trucks. I was just standing there and everything went dark. When I woke up, I was lying on my back facing the ceiling of the truck. Two weeks had gone by, so I thought I better go and see the boss. He said he was glad to see me he wanted us to talk. Well it didn't take me long to get his drift, he was firing me. He didn't think I was big or strong enough to do the job. I thanked him for being candid and I left his office. I didn't feel bad about being fired, because I knew I was not right for that job.

Worked As a Pastoral Assistant—April 2, 2002

After the warehouse job didn't work out, I thought that maybe I would do better with an indoor less physical job. I knew the Pastor from working in the warehouse. The Pastor worked at a church that had a seventy-bed facility for an alcohol rehabilitation center for men. The warehouse was used as a work place for the men in rehabilitation.

I setup an appointment to see the Pastor and discuss my illness, background, and some the ideas I had. He knew my background in Biblical studies. We seemed to hit it off right from the beginning. He told me the job didn't come with a paycheck. I told him that was all right; I was trying to stay active and continue to work on my recovery from a nervous system shutdown. He said I appeared to have enough training and experience with traumatic issue that I would be of assistance to the men in rehabilitation.

As time passed, I assisted the Pastor with his duties, upgraded the computers at the church, and started a resume service for the graduates seeking employment. I did a woodworking to create personalized crosses for the graduates of the program. The Pastor notice that I could only work about three hours before becoming so weary, that I would have to lie down on the couch in the Pastoral study and sleep for about three hours. After one of these three-hour sleep periods, I woke up and heard heavenly music. I wondered if I was dead, but the Pastor took off his headsets and asked me if I slept well. I asked him why he was wearing the headsets. He told me he was writing his sermon and my snoring broke his concentration. I apologized for the ruckus, we laughed, and he said he didn't mind. The Pastor could see that my three-hour work and three hour sleep was an endless cycle. He could see that this would be a big problem working at a regular job. I told him I just kept on trying, waiting for the day I would return to being my normal self. I worked for the Pastor for about nine months. Then I began having problems with my memory again. I could not determine what I was doing. I was walking around in a daze. He suggested that I try working at one of the thrift stores and see how I do there. It was a sad parting because we really liked working together and doing things for others. I told him when I couldn't help myself it was impossible to help others. He understood. I was not depressed after this job, I just pressed forward to the next job.

Worked In a Thrift Store—April 3, 2002

Working at the thrift store was another volunteer job. This job was more physical than working with the Pastor, but I didn't have to figure things out. All I had to do was put items in their proper place on the shelves. I thought, surely I could do this job. I could not remember where to place the items. The work hours were from 7:30 am to 5 pm. I could only work until 1 pm. I was not able to sleep every three hours. After a month or so, I had to quit. I was very depressed. I felt like my recovery was going backwards.

Worked With Co-Worker—April 5, 2002

A friend, that knew me from my previous computer jobs, asked if I wanted to work for her. At this point, I was open to anything. After the first day on the job, she saw how unstable I was and never assigned me any work. I guess that was a kind way of telling me, that she didn't want me working with her customers. I think my actions and mannerisms were too much for her to handle.

I was depressed for well over six months. I just stayed at home and seemed to drift off into trances all day. I could not seem to get my mind to function correctly.

Worked On Two Paper Routes—April 5, 2002

I worked for a major newspaper company delivering papers to individual homes. It seemed to me that this would be a simple task. I couldn't remember the addresses of the houses that were to receive papers. My mind would invert the house numbers, which completely confused me. As we went through the paper route, I couldn't remember what streets we had delivered papers. This was in the middle of winter. There was at least eight inches of snow on the ground. Since I was having problems, my wife thought she would go with me and see if she could improve my situation. She helped me deliver papers for about a month.

One morning, at 3 am, we were delivering papers using an older model 1977 Blazer with oversized large tires. We were throwing the newspapers, wrapped in plastic, from each of our side windows. I was driving the truck with my right arm and throwing papers with my left arm. We were traveling about fifteen miles an hour, the flashers were on, and we were driving in the center of the neighborhood streets. We were on a street that was not very well lighted. My wife was throwing papers from her side. I threw a paper out my side and I never saw the paper go towards the house. A few seconds later, we heard a loud boom, as the Sunday paper hit the roof of the truck. Looking at each other, we started to laugh! We stopped the truck in the middle of the road. It was snowing like crazy. We got out of the truck and we were still laughing. Since the truck had big tires, we couldn't see the newspaper on the roof beneath four inches of snow. We each got a Sunday paper and stood in the doorway of the truck trying to push the newspaper off the roof. As if we didn't have enough problems, here came the police with lights a flashing.

The police got out of their car and approached us cautiously. They asked what our problem was. My wife and I were still laughing about the newspaper landing on the roof of the truck. We were sure that the police didn't understand what was going on. They see two nuts in the middle of the street, pushing something back and forth on the roof of a truck, at 3 am in the morning. I explained that I had a problem with my arm and that I threw a newspaper on the top of the truck. The police officer was busy explaining the dangers of leaving our truck in the middle of the road during a snowstorm. We agreed with him, while we were laughing and working to get the newspaper off the roof. The police returned to their car, turned off their lights, and slowly disappeared in the snow. Now, we started laughing about going to jail for throwing a Sunday newspaper on the roof of a truck. We were not successful delivering all of the newspapers, but we had fun!

This is a funny story, but I had lost all control of my left arm. Between problems with my memory and my arm, we stopped delivering papers that night.

Medical Transcriptions Course—April 5, 2002

I tried working on the first and second book of a medical transcription course. I read it, but I could not remember anything at all. My wife had to cancel the course for me.

Operation on Arm—April 3, 2002

During the spring of that year, the problems with my left arm continued to get worse. I had constant pain in my wrist and the Orthopedics doctor had me wear braces for a while to determine if I had carpal tunnel. I again went to a Neurologist to have the nerve connections from my hand to my shoulder checked. I told him that I couldn't feel three of my fingers. The results of his test showed that the nerves between my elbow and bicep were severed. The Orthopedics Surgeon performed surgery on my left elbow and on the inside of by bicep. The operation was successful. I had to go to therapy to restore the physical use of my arm. It took over a year and a half for the nerves to begin working again. Now, I can feel my fingers.

Worked At the Dog Kennel—April 6, 2002

Once I was able to feel my fingers again, I thought it was time to try another job. I liked animals, particularly dogs. My wife and I saw that there were some job openings at the County Dog Kennel. She applied to work directly with the dogs in the kennel area. I applied for a job in the administrative area since I could type on a computer. A few days later, my wife got a call and she took the job. I sat at home feeling depressed, but hopeful. About two weeks later, I got a call for an interview. They explained that the job was answering phone inquiries and entering information in the computer. I thought this would be easy, so I accepted the job.

I worked there for two and a half months. I was having problems dealing with the people that called on the phone. They were yelling, screaming, and cursing me up one side and down the other. I would just hang up on them. After my background, I wasn't going to put up with any bodies crap. It seemed as though the supervisor called me into her office at least once a day to discuss problems between customers and me on the phone. Some days, I went in her office more than once. She said, "I should be pleasant and kind on the phone even if the caller was not." I just told her, "All right." I thought to myself, "There was no way that I was going to let a bunch of rude lowlife idiots run over me." I found myself telling these people in a pleasant way, where to stick it. I never used a bad word. I guess people are not ready to be told where to stick it, when they are rude.

See, Dr. Wadeson explained to me that my PTSD condition was no ones business except mine. I thought, "Yea, I'm not a danger to anyone, I'm just a nut case." "I don't think it's against the law to be a nut. I see them everywhere." When I filled out my application, I didn't say anything about my condition. The supervisor said that I acted strangely different from the other employees. She said she couldn't exactly put her finger on the problem. I should watch my step. I walked out of her office thinking, "If you only knew."

While I was working, they had a screen saver running on the computer terminal. Sometimes it would bounce words around, draw graphic lines, or draw pipes on the screen. Well, these screen saver images would cause me to go into a trance. I didn't hear anything that was going on in the room. I didn't hear the phones ringing either. Two young girls got extremely upset with me. They would curse at me for not answering the phones, but I really didn't hear a word they said. One day the girls got so mad, they began verbally assaulting me in a way they never did before. It would have made a sailor blush. This time I was listening and heard every word. I was so upset I started stuttering and could not remember what to say on the phone. I was in a real panic and didn't know what to do. I stood up and said with a loud voice, "I don't have to take this crap!" Then, I walked out. That was my last day working at the dog kennel.

I've learned that no matter what may happen to me, I just keep going on. Keep on trying and never give up.

After this job experience, I was in a deep depression for about another year. I spent my days sitting on the couch in a trance.

7

Continued Gradual Recovery 2001–2002

Deep Depression—January—February 2001

During January and February of 2001, I cannot remember anything except I was in a deep depression. I had been in a depression for so long, I didn't know any other way of feeling. I hadn't written in a journal for quite a while. The year 1998, was the last papers and journal that I found, while looking through the upstairs closet. It seems to me that the years 1999 and 2000 were my most extremely depressed years. No about of control or medication could bring me out of this condition.

In 2001, Dr. Wadeson asked me to start keeping a journal again. I hadn't written things or events in my journal for a couple of reasons. First, I had been very depressed and hadn't felt that anything was getting better. I was stuck where I was, with no recovery in site, and there was no one that could get me out of this prison. I tried to write, but every time I wrote, I would end up writing the same stuff repeatedly. Second, I had resigned myself to being disabled with PTSD for the rest of my life. I also, had a fear of allowing anyone to read my journal or see the crazy things going through my mind. I had been plagued with hallucinations, visions, and images (pictures) in my mind continually.

My Thinking Began To Change—March 2001

Let me continue with March 2001; my thinking began to change about this time. I don't really know why things started to change.

My wife injured herself at work. She had injured the alignment of her back and had shooting pains in her leg. She needed to take it easy for a while. During this time, I was getting worse. I spent my time sleeping and sitting in the living room, caught up in a trance. My wife would ask me, what am I looking at? All I could say was, I don't know!

I didn't know at the time, I was viewing Intrusive Memories (IM). I had no idea anything like that transpired. If a person observes or experiences something long enough, the happening is no longer new or unfamiliar. Like a person that has poor vision, doesn't realize it until the doctor shows him what clear site looks like. The reaction is Wow. I didn't know things could look this clear.

It was with all the things controlling my mind. All I could seem to tell my doctor was how sad, tired, angry, upset, and overwhelmed I was. I did my very best to describe what was happening to me. I didn't know the words to describe the symptoms to the doctor. I told him I felt helpless and hopeless. Nothing really mattered, because I couldn't feel anything. I thought I would be stuck like this forever.

My wife suggested I get more help. Get any kind of help such as, inpatient, outpatient, group home, or group therapy. Something—just do something! She couldn't stand this anymore! She felt she couldn't go on like this!

This struck a great fear in me! Would she leave me? She was the last friend I had. All of the other people I knew had faded away. I had no family and no friends. What would I lose my wife next? I was struck with terror! I was frantic! Just writing this in my journal, I have a crushing headache, my neck is so tight I cannot turn my head, and my whole body is shaking. My palms are sweating and my head is bobbing like a little display dog in the back window of a car. Boy, this is so hard for me to write!

From 1995 to 2001, I have refused to enter a psycho ward of a hospital, because I didn't think I'd ever get out. I had a very hard time explaining things to Dr. Wadeson during private therapy sessions. This time when I went to see Dr. Wadeson, I had a new incentive to take some kind of action. I didn't want my wife to leave! I explained my situation to Dr. Wadeson and he immediately placed me in a men's therapy group. I was telling him that the group session would be great and inside I was scared to death. Up to this time, I was so overwhelmed with shame I felt that it was impossible for me to tell what I called the family secrets, in any kind of public forum. I had no idea of what to expect when attending a group session.

I have always prayed and asked all of the obvious questions. I prayed for guidance and strength to endure this illness. I haven't heard an answer yet. Now, I see another great high mountain with snow and ice on its peaks. This of course it the challenge of facing a group session and trying to tear these devastating traumatic events from my mind and telling them to total strangers. I knew the snow and ice on that mountain came with an extremely bitter cold wind. This would be a rough challenge.

Started Group Therapy—April 2001

The group therapy began to take effect. The other men told of hard things they had experienced. As the months went by, I felt a kind of kinship with them. As I told them of my experiences, no one said a word. Their mouths dropped open and they had no idea of what to say. Dr. Wadeson was quick to pick up the pace of the session and move on to another subject. The one thing I received from each of them was empathy and usually a statement such as; I don't think I could have lived through all your experiences.

Concentration Practice—May—June—July 2001

Dr. Wadeson changed half of my medications. I didn't notice any difference at all. I thought, here we go again another dead end. Dr. Wadeson asked me to work on trying to concentrate on different issues. I thought to myself, "Right, I have trouble concentrating on just shaving." Even though I had my doubts, I spent my time thinking of things I could concentrate.

I hadn't listened to the radio since I became ill in 1995. I tried to listen to the radio, but there was an endless stream of information. The radio was too much for my mind to handle. I tried to watch TV from time to time, but even a movie or show had too many characters, plots, places, and pictures for me to remember what was going on. Again, I tried to watch the TV. I searched all of the cable stations on TV. I thought this was a real maze of information. My head was spinning after only 15 minutes of watching TV. After weeks of searching the channels, I found that I could remember the number of the last channel I was watching. I told Dr. Wadeson with excitement and he said, "Good—keep on going."

Weeks had passed and I found a channel that had country videos. I thought that since the songs were only two or three minutes long, maybe I could us this. Great, maybe I've found something that was short enough that I could concentrate on. Well, I started to concentrate, but I lost it many times. I could not tell the beginning of the song from the end. After only a short time into a song—I had to leave the living room and go to the kitchen. Just to get away from everything and relax quietly by myself. I had to get away from all of the noise and information that was flooding my mind. I actually got a headache from all of the pictures. I thought I would explode. It was as if I had a thousand people screaming at me all at the same time.

With clinched fists, I sat on the couch in the living room. I went through one video, forcing myself to watch the complete video to the end. I made it. With pounding head and tight neck, I went back into the kitchen to have a cigarette. My mind raced ever faster. I wandered if this flood of information going through my mind would ever stop.

I was thinking back to when my brain shutdown at the beginning of this illness. I surely didn't want to push things that far and have to starting all over again. I had never traveled this road before. There were many questions and doubts in my mind. The only thing I was sure of was the instructions from Dr. Wadeson, "Try to concentrate." I thought he must know what he's asking me to do. He must know how I'm feeling. He must know how painful this process is for me to accomplish. All of these thoughts kept running through my mind. I had to trust someone and I chose Dr. Wadeson. I made up my mind that what ever he asked me to do, whether it was hard or easy I would try my best to accomplish the request. Trusting someone was extremely hard for me. I never trusted in anyone completely, except for my wife.

Within a month, that would be June of 2001, I could sit and watch country videos for an hour or so. I reported my progress to Dr. Wadeson, he said, "That's good." He told me to work on watching a movie. He added, "Let's keep going." I thought to myself, "Don't you hate it when a doctor seems so matter of fact about things. It's like they know something we don't." No matter I did as he requested.

I noticed that all throughout my recovery, everything had been done in baby steps. Sometimes my wife didn't even know about or see my progress. That was depressing to me. I had talked to Dr. Wadeson about this and he told me, "Not to worry about it." He added, "Don't even bring the subject up with anyone, all of these small steps will be seen soon enough." "Just keep your mind on concentrating." I felt as a child coming home from school with an 'A' on my paper and then the teacher says, "Wait until report card day to tell your parents."

Ok, the next step was to watch a complete movie. I chose an action video, because that is my favorite type of movie to watch. I was thinking with my upbeat attitude, a video I liked, and my drive to succeed this would be an easy task. This was not so! I tried! I put on the video and started to watch. Sometime in the very beginning of the movie, I became so overwhelmed from pictures, words, and the storyline. I throw up! I was seeing that there was an unmistakable connection between the mental and physical experiences.

Well, it was time for a cigarette, so off to the kitchen I went. I had to contemplate the dilemma I was facing. I didn't want to give up. After thinking for a while, I decided to try some show that was thirty-minutes to an hour in length. I scanned the channels one by one. I didn't know how to use the electronic TV guide yet. Finally, I came across a show about lawyers. This show had some action, but low intensity. This show didn't have fast action, loud special effect, or a complicated story line.

I spent a few days watching different thirty-minute shows. It was another month before I could watch a complete movie. After watching a movie, I had to go to sleep for two to three hours. I could hardly function at all. I was completely physically worn out. I couldn't think any more. No, I couldn't remember anything about the movie.

My wife and I went to the bookstore to see if we could find a book on PTSD. This was the first time that I felt I could try to read some information about my illness. I had not been able to read books or comprehend what was in them. I had to read the same paragraph repeatedly with no luck. We only found two books in the store that had any information related to stress or trauma. We bought the books and began reading. I took the book about overwhelming stress. This book also spoke on the subject of PTSD. I could only read one page and have to put the book down. My mind was overcome by the about of information those few words conveyed.

Having a Blackout—August 2001

On August 5, 2001, I came down to the kitchen table at about 5 am. I usually start the coffee brewing, but this morning I sat at the table, started to smoke a cigarette—closed my eyes and—All I could see in my mind was black. I opened and closed my eyes and still all I could see is black—time went by—suddenly, I heard a loud pop inside my head and then Images of all my life began flowing across my mind! The speed of the picture movie was so fast; I became sick to my stomach.

As I write this down, my whole body is shaking—not just my hands. My insides feel as though they are turning over! (Even now, as I type this in on April 6, 2002, my whole body is shaking!) I talked to my wife about this and she was amazed! We both said this seemed like what happened in 1995 when I first became ill. I don't know when these things will end, if ever. I have been quite upset inside ever since this event occurred. The rest of the day, my wife said, "I turned conversations around." She was talking about who was in a movie and I thought she was talking about what was in the movie. Later I turned the information of an event around when I was talking to my brother in law. I am becoming extremely distressed!

Limbs on Fire—August 2001

On August 17, 2001, I made a note to myself to discuss this heat problem with Dr. Wadeson.

This kind of personal subject matter I hate to reveal about myself or even write it down in this journal. I have had to work through being able to express any kind of feelings. I still have not become able to vocalize my feelings. Only since December of 2001, have I been able to write down my feelings and provide them to any doctor. Now, I am in the process of providing this information to the public.

When I said I wasn't feeling well, I described it this way: Something comes over me, heat rushes through my body, and every limb is on fire. Sometimes I break out into a sweat. I become so angry; I could explode or kill someone. Usually, this feeling goes away after thirty minutes or so. Then, I cannot believe anything happened at all. The same thing happened on the 16th Thursday. This time the anger was caused by my inability to make my brother-in-law and my wife understand what I was trying to say. In my mind, I was able to think the words I wanted to say. The problem comes in when I try to get my brain to give the right words to my mouth. For me this is frustrating to say the least. If I am in a group of people, I become so overwhelmed by the all the words from all the people, I can't speak at all. If I don't remove myself from the location, I go into a trance. That occurs when my brain shuts down.

Passed Out Due To Trauma—September 2001

The events of September 11, 2001 caused me a great deal of distress. I passed out while watching the news. These events caused an increase in the number of Intrusive Memories (IM). They completely controlled my mind. I was totally disabled for the beginning of the month of September. I slept a lot, I couldn't think straight, I was confused, and I felt like I was not even in this world. I was in the world built by my mind. I saw hundreds of moving pictures flashing in my mind and I could not control anything about what was happening. I was struggling desperately to find a way to explain what was happening to Dr. Wadeson, so he could help me.

Towards the end of the month, my mind started to change. Where before I wasn't interested in anything, now I was overwhelmed by a need to find out everything I could about PTSD. I had to know if there was any possibility of something I could do to help myself. I wanted to know if anyone else had been able to work his or her way out of this illness or were others stuck like me. I looked at this in two ways. One view was of fear of what I would find. The other was an extreme interest in what I might learn to help myself.

Alaska Died—October—November 2001

On October 3, 2001, my faithful companion for over ten years, ALASKA died. She was a red and white, eighty-pound Siberian husky. This sent me into a deep depression. She was my one source of strength and constant companion throughout my years of illness. Loosing her, hurt me more than all the effects of PTSD ever could. It wasn't until February of 2002, that I was able to write down my feeling about her death. October and November of 2001, I was not able to write anything. I didn't have the will or the drive to write or do anything, except eat a little and sleep a lot. I wrote a tribute to her and I have placed it at the head of this book.

Research Began—December 2001

In December 2001, I was overcome with a strong desire to read everything I could about PTSD. I read everything I could find on the Internet, books, pamphlets, and magazine articles. During the following months, I was driven to write everything I knew about PTSD. Through reading about PTSD, I learned the words Dr. Wadeson understood about the disease. Now, I had to find a way of writing down what was happening in my mind and body, so he could help me. I felt a drive inside of me, anger with myself, which I did not know how to explain the phenomena that were going on in my brain. I had a mission, to make Dr. Wadeson understand!

Dr. Wadeson and I decided that all of the information I had written should be compiled into a book, to assist others affected by mental illness. This book might be thought of as just another tool, which will allow others to explain their unique situations to their own doctors.

A Book Was Born—December 28, 2001—April 15, 2002

I wrote the book, "I Cry for Help!" This is not intended to be a medical book. This book is my own personal chronicle, which provides some understanding of the mysteries of PTSD. In my situation, all of the adverse affects of abuse, trauma, combat trauma, stress, overwork, caused PTSD over study, working days, and going to school at night. In addition, this book shows through actual real life events, a way of learning about the decease, and coping skills to live in a more understandable world.

There is NOT a cure for PTSD at present, knowledge, coping skills, and medicine are what is currently available.

I do not want to exclude prescribed medications by a Physiatrist. However, I'm not a doctor; I can't about that subject. See your Physiatrist.

I know that I am only able to function today by using many medications. Having a Psychiatrist treating you is necessary!

8

Accomplishment before PTSD

Military Service—Mar. 12, 2002

While living at my birth mothers house, my schedule was to attend school in the morning and work a minimum wage job for about six hours each afternoon. As the year progressed, my decision to join the armed forces was firmed up in my mind. This would allow me to leave my hometown, all my problems behind, and start a new life in a new place. My goals were to experience travel, go anywhere the military had in mind, and see what the world had to offer. Additional goals were to increase my education, learn a viable trade or a profession to start me on life's journey. Like most eighteen year olds, I had the readiness to go anywhere but here, so that I could leave my childhood behind, and hit the open road.

While in the Navy Recruiters Office in Washington, D.C. to sign up for the Navy in April of 1968, there were many people below the office burning cars, building, and rioting throughout the streets of the city. The assassination of Martin Luther King in the south sent a chilling ripple across the United States of sympathy and the people took to the streets in protest. Being a youth, I was not sure what live was all about.

There was a national uprising-taking place, at college and university campuses concerning our involvement in the Vietnam War. Many young service men went on two-year combat tours. Like them I took my turn and received the, Vietnam Combat Service Medal eight times, Vietnam Service Medal two times, National Defense Medal, Presidential Unit Citation Medal, Marine Unit Accommodation Medal, and an Honorable Discharge.

During my four-year tour of duty from '68 to '72, the opportunity to visit more than twelve allied countries around the world was very satisfying. Attending a number of schools, my goal of having a trade was fulfilled. After four disciplined years, the challenges of civilian life appear very bright.

A red MG Midget convertible was the give I bought for my duty in the service. Four months of vacation to tour the U.S. was the other goal that sustained my imagination during this time of transition. After my vacation, going back to work was my next goal.

U.S. Government with Navy DOD—Mar. 15, 2002

With great excitement obtaining a Radio Telecommunications Operator job working for the Navy, under the Department of Defense was another goal accomplished. There was a military and civilian side to separate military messages from civilian messages. When referencing to two sides, it was exactly that, a door divided the two sections. The door had a small ten-inch mail slot cut in the door to relay message.

I met a cute young girl with dark hair and hazel eyes, through the slot in the door. We often communicated through that door for over a year. Sending my personal message to her, she would respond with a message through the door. This was a unique relationship. She had the cutest face and those hazel eyes mesmerized me. One day I sent her a message asking her out on a date and two months later on June 29, 1973, we were married. She is still my wife and a grandmother. I believe that finding each other through that doorway was the most important accomplishment of my life. We still kept our message sending alive at home by writing daily in a spiral notebook. My grandson says this is a very weird way to me a girl. He may be correct! Where was email when we needed it? In September of 1976, we were expecting our first child. Being concerned about finances, I began a long series of attending school at night that lasted twenty years.

Civilian Computer Contracting—Mar. 15, 2002

Spend two to two and a half years at different companies allowed me to obtain knowledge about many computers seemed to be a good strategy. Continuing that strategy, I learned knowledge about computer software application, programming languages, and control protocols. With knowledge of different computer disciplines set me up for job security to support my family.

From March of '77 to '95, I steadily moved through the ranks from Junior Programmer to Computer Scientist Section Manager increasing my responsibilities of personnel and systems.

I took over as Section Manager, after by boss at age forty-five had a heart attach. The doctor told him to get out of this business or the stress would kill him. He retired. I only stayed in the position for three years and I could not take the continual presser from the job. During this complete period, we worked on Critical Systems for the Navy, which brought a level of stress maintain these systems.

As in many job there are uncontrolled power used in excess by supervisors at higher levels. I'm not complaining nor standing on a soapbox, I'm just showing how irresponsible some bosses can be when they have unchecked power. This causes undue hardships and extreme stress on both employees and their families. I learned about the "Old Boy's Club," I guess it could be referred to as the (OBC). Learning that there are always a few people within an organization government or civilian that have been around since an organization or project got off the grounds, which are granted special powers. All of the personnel were about the same age and worked very hard together to get everything started. Without his or her efforts, no one else would be working there at present. I can see why this can happen. The problem comes in, when the members of this little excusive 'Old Boy's Club,' ignore the irresponsible actions and undue cruelties committed, condoned, and covered up by the others in the group. I tried, in vain, for three years to reason with this group of individuals. This is when the labels were announced, that I was, "Not a team player," "Rocking the boat," "Didn't understand how the political system works," and "Creating too many waves." I'm sure you've heard them all. I also, saw irregularities having to do with actions with personnel, labor hour reporting practices, leave allocations; promotions and appreciations ignored or refused, arbitrary development schedule changes, and unacceptable working schedules. I called my bosses on all of these matters. I was talked to very gentle, they said I didn't understand the big picture. They said I was thinking to low level and down to the details. What a bunch of crap! I left after there were no additional improvements I could possibly contribute.

Since I had both a military and an extensive communications background, another civilian contracting company accepted me. This company was based in Arlington, Virginia. They were contracted to the U.S. Army Criminal Investigation Division (CID), to support the worldwide communications requirements, utilizing the Internet as a network base. I worked for this company from 1993-94. I maintained, updated, and performed trouble shooting for an Ethernet Local Area Network (LAN) housed within a six-floor build. The microcomputers on this LAN utilized both Windows and Unix Operating Systems. Again, I traveled all over the Northeast and Midwest U.S. at a moments notice.

One of the most exciting projects was preparing a Unix System with satellite Internet connectivity, which was delivered to the U.S. Army troops stationed in Somalia, Africa. They had a unique problem, once the system was installed in an S10 Blazer used for mobility. The problem occurred about the same time every night, Somalia time. I had written software that would maintain a signal of contact with the entire CID computer system around the world. My Signal Ping System would log the Somalia computer down everyday about the same time in Arlington, Virginia. I would contact them by phone to assist them in reactivating the system. With some analysis on their part, they found out that the kids were digging up the communications cable and cut it up into four-foot sections. We didn't have a clue as to why they cutting up the cable. CID Somalia advised us that the children were making jump ropes out of the cable. We decided that the most viable solution to the problem was to send a roll of cable to Somalia as soon as possible. CID Somalia invited the children to come to the Blazer Communications site and receive free jump ropes. Communications was restored and performed well for the rest of the Somalia operations. The children were all getting stronger using their new jump ropes.

From 1994-95, I was contracted to the National Science Foundation in Falls Church, Virginia. During this year, my responsibilities as the Internet Post Master included System Administration, Email, and Personnel Account for all of the NSF Government Employees. All of the systems that I was responsible for were UNIX based computers. This was a high visibility position with an extreme amount of stress. I worked at home via a dialup Internet connection. I had both Windows and UNIX systems at my home, which I purchased so that I would not have to drive to the NSF during the night. I worked from home in support of the NSF three to four hours every night.

In March of 1995, I took a job as a System Administrator with a New York base company named PenCom. They flew me to Austin, Texas for eight interviews by their managers; additional interviews over the phone to New York city, San Francisco, California, and Washington, D.C. I was hired as a Systems Administrator for UNIX base systems. I was one of team of three employees sent to a site located in Laurel, Maryland. Our contract was with the Internal Revenue Service. I was responsible for over 300 Computer Systems. They had a shift work schedule, so our service was 24 hours a day 7 days a week. We all were responsible to satisfy the needs of over 1,200 IRS employees. That proved to be too much stress for me to handle. On May 10, 1995, I had a nervous breakdown. On June 16, 1995, I was fired because I did not have any more leave. They said my work was excellent. They said to give them a call when I recover. I am still in the process of recovering.

Too Many Responsibilities—Extreme Stress—Mar. 18, 2002

From 1977-1995, I traveled all over the U.S. on a moments notice, went to school both day and night, worked both day and night via dialup and internet connections installed at my home, and my work responsibilities never really stopped. I was upset and despondent, but I always chalked it up to having an important job came with additional responsibilities. I surely was not going to give up, quit, complain, or shirk my responsibilities according to the contract. It always had the phrase; "the incumbent shall provide all required service within four hours." I saw that statement, but I didn't think it would always be my turn. I thought I just had to reach down deeper inside myself to give all I had. When I had a nervous system, shutdown on May 10, 1995, I knew I had given my all. I had no more to give. For the last nine years now, my family has paid the price for my mistake in judgment. I lost my job, and then my wife had to retire early from her job to take care of me. To make ends meet, we had to use all of our saving and 401k retirement funds. We sold our boat, truck, and car to try to stay afloat. We had no more funds, so finally we had to sell our house. Remember, I was making close to $70,000 and my wife was making $30,000 a year. I had a long-term disability insurance plan to take care of any major medical problems. When we submitted our claim, we found out that the insurance didn't cover any type of mental breakdown.

9

Our Life Before PTSD

I went to see Dr. Wadeson for my regular appointment on April 18, 2002. He asked me to write about how my life was before I became ill with PTSD. I told him I would do my best. I thought, "Before PTSD, that part of my life was a mess also."

I served four years Honorably and Decorated in the U.S. Navy as a communications radioman. I served my first year in the Vietnam War. I returned to the United States where I attended communications school for nine months. I served my next year or so under the Admiral of ComCorTron8; we were a communications readiness-testing group. We traveled from ship to ship determining if the crews were ready for war. It was exciting duty traveling with the Admiral; I had the opportunity to visit about thirteen different counties attached by three different oceans.

I had two extraordinary events happen to me while I was with this command. The first one happened when we enter the port at Naples, Italy. I received an emergency phone call. I was called to the Executive Officers cabin. Much to my surprise, it was a call from my birth mother, telling me that my sister had been kidnapped and the police could not find her. I was visibly shaken by the news! I told her I would call her back. I conferred with the Executive Officer and the Operations Officer I worked under and asked them if this was grounds for emergency leave. The Operations Officer said that I was in no condition to continue my duties. They granted me thirty days leave to work the matter out. I returned the phone call and told her I would be home as soon as possible. They transferred me to a ship that was in the same taskforce, Stateside in Newport, Rhode Island. That way I could go on leave and just return to the ship in Rhode Island. This ship would be leaving for the Mediterranean Sea by the time I returned.

When I returned to the States, my birth mother had a story that was all mixed up. I couldn't understand what the problem was! This was my first indication that there was something very wrong with my mothers thinking. I said I'd never return to my father and stepmother's house, but this seemed necessary. I called my father and he told me that the man that kidnapper my sister was at his house, right now. I didn't understand—what was a kidnapper doing at his house. Aren't these people supposed to be in jail or something! I told him that I would drive to his house, if we would give me the directions. I hadn't slept in about two days.

When I got there, I was more astonished than upset. They told me a very confusing story. I talked with the kidnapper and my parent all night long. This is the best of the story I can remember. This is a real mind juggler. Somehow, this man was in love with my sister and she went away with him by her own free will. Ok, that means no kidnapping. They wanted to get married, but the parents didn't agree, because of their age differences. That's the reason they ran away together.

I really couldn't believe it. I was sitting there after traveling from Naples Italy; it is 5 am, after talking all night, to find out that this is a love event! I wished them well and I went home. Now, I really needed the well-deserved thirty days of leave.

Remember, I told you there were two extraordinary events that happened to me. Well, here is the other story.

I returned from leave and reported to my ship in Newport, Rhode Island. I thought it was nice changing ships and working with new crews of sailors. On this ship, I fit in well. I was promoted to an "At Sea Supervisor." That meant that I had qualified to run everything in the radio shack by myself. This is a proficiency rating. No money came with this promotion. While I was on this ship, I became good friends with the Radio Chief. We would talk about how things were back home, our families, and about his kids. This friendship grew until the Chief was someone I could confide in about personal matters that concerned me.

Each day everyone assembled for the most anticipated event, which was mail call. The crew always looked forward to that stateside connection. I seemed to start receiving more and more letters from home. I wasn't concerned by the quantity of letters. I intensely disturbed by the content of these letters. Time went by and I had a stack of letters. I didn't know what to think about what was in the letters. I kept this to myself; I surely didn't want to divulge the troubling stories to my fellow crewmembers. I began to dread mail call. I knew it would be just more of the same. It was a few months before I couldn't stand it anymore. The pressure was too much for me to bear. I made an appointment to speak to the Radio Chief, that's like my top sergeant.

I asked him to read a letter and then tell me whom he thought it came from. He took his time and said this is from your girl friend. I gave him a couple more letters. He read them and said, "These are from your girl friend. She sounds like she really misses you. Right? I told him, "NO!" He asked, "What do you mean?" I took a deep breath and after a long pause, I told him, "All of these letters were from my birth mother!" He said, "What? These are love letters!" I said, "I know." I broke down and started crying like a baby. Here I was twenty-two years old and in front of my Chief, I break down. I was humiliated and confused. I was a fighting warrior, ready for combat at anytime. This was destroying me! This was my second indication that there was something very wrong with my mothers thinking.

I asked the Chief for his help. I needed to transfer to a place where my family could not contact me. I told him of the special communications group that the CNO of the Navy was creating. He looked at me and said, "yes." I told him, I wanted to volunteer for Group F44 immediately. He said, "We'd sleep on it and then review this in the morning." I couldn't sleep; I just wanted to get away from Italy.

The next morning the Chief said he would fix things up and I'd be on my way to Group F44 based in Vietnam. Within two-weeks, I was traveling to Survival Training in Coronado, California. Training was about six week. I was hopped on a plane bound for Vietnam. I spent my final year in the Vietnam War, serving under the CNO of the Navy. The one thing I've never told anyone before was, that I felt so low about this letter problem, I actually hoped that I would die in the war! I had no desire in returning home. I didn't care about my own safety. I never endangered others. I had nerves of steel; I figured that if they shot me, they shot me. The group of us in F44 had a saying or a type of philosophy we used. I may sound corny, but we used what ever worked. The saying went like this:

If you hear bullets and shells going, off,
    Then you're ok, because you're not dead.
If you are hit and feel pain. Then you're still ok,
    Call for a medic, because you're not dead.
If you are hit by a shell and feel no pain,
    Then you're ok, because you're dead.

When I returned to the United States, or as the Vietnam Veterans called it, "Going Back to the World" the attitudes of the American people had completely changed. Everyone was against the War.

All of the military people I came back with seemed to be regular normal people. "After finally arriving at a real town, everyone cuts up a bit and we went wild!

It's the only place to let down your guard, at least for a few hours." All of us seemed to have the same type of attitudes. "Jump in our face and we all kill you!" We had all been through hell and survived ok. We all had a bond, which I had never know before or since the war. Everyone was trained to work as one unit, one complete person. Everyone knew how to anticipate the next persons move. There was a surety that someone was always watching your back. Never did we feel alone. When we came back from the war, they didn't show us how to be deprogrammed from four years of military life. Nor did they show us how to re-enter civilian society. We had been taught deadly things to do automatically. No thinking about it, you do it or you die. There was one aspect of returning home that I had never thought of, we were not the same as the so-called normal people in the U.S. Each of us, for the first time, would be walking point alone. It would take each of us over six years to acclimate ourselves to a society which was based on self-control. We had been trained to execute commands automatically. This would be our next big challenge.

After I returned from Vietnam, it was 1972; I took a trip to Newport, Rhode Island. To visit a friend from Vietnam and see how he was doing. After the visit with him and his girlfriend, I left and went to the beach. I was extremely depressed, I thought, I couldn't take this anymore! I took a bottle of pills to kill myself! I fell asleep thinking this is the end of this letter mess! I woke up the next morning on the beach and I felt as though nothing happened. I thought I should be sick or something. I guess it wasn't to be! I never got over the letters and I was too embarrassed to ask my birth mother anything about them.

I didn't stay home long. I packed up my stuff and I hit the open road. During three years in the service, I was paying for a new red and black convertible 1972 MG-Midget. It was waiting for me when I arrived home. I didn't seem to stay in any one place to long. I went and visited people I knew and just did some traveling up and down the east coast of the U.S. I wanted to see all that I had missed.

I went to visit a relative's house in New Jersey to determine if I could get a job there. I only was going to stay for two weeks, and then I was going to leave, so I would not cause any domestic problems. Well, I put in many applications for jobs, but only one job called me. I thought ok, I'd try anything once.

Boy, was this a different kind of job. The advertisement said it was a canning factory. My relative said that there were many canning factories in New Jersey and across the river in Philadelphia, Pa. I made an appointment to see the boss and drove out to the canning plant. When I arrived it, was lunchtime and I observed a large group of people going across the street to a bar. I didn't think too much about it at the time. I went in, found where the offices were and the secretary said the boss would be right with me. He came out and greeted me, read my application, and said this is not a job for you. I wander about what he said. I really need a job and I told him so. He started talking to me about the Navy and said he was a retired Chief. He said you're too intelligent for this job. Then, I asked him what the big deal about this job is? He said come on back here and I'll show you what you'll be doing.

He had me really thinking about what this job had in store for me. Well, he showed all of the production processing lines and the cans were just a flying on their way to be boxed up for shipping. Trucks were rolling in and out and that looked all normal to me. Then, he took me behind some hanging clear plastic dividers. Man, what a smell there was in that room! My eyes started to water. I asked him smartly, what is that smell! He said you'd see. He continued to show me all the machines and clear plastic pipes about eight to ten inches in diameter. They ran from one end of building to the other. I ask him timidly, what's moving up there in those pipes. He answers swiftly, that's dog food, sailor boy! Ok, now I was getting it, this was a dog food factory. I was thinking in terms of a vegetable canning factory. Soup? Beans? No, this was the worst smelling dog food in the world! I was thinking when I find out the name of this stuff, my dog is not even coming close to this stuff! A dog could die from eating this stuff! While the boss was showing me around, he was talking to the different workers. I thought I'd look around. I was busy watching how this one big plastic tube branched into additional tubes and then they went through the wall to somewhere. I just couldn't get over the red gooey ooze that was flowing through that pipe! Man, that ooze in the pipe was gross!

Now, the boss said sailor boy, come this way. We went through another barrier of plastic dividers. I thought I would die; the smell was so bad it astounded me! I'm talking about a smell that was so thick; you would swear you could touch it with your hands. By this time, I looked at the Chief, and he smiled at me as he said nice work environment isn't it! My eyes were watering, I couldn't respond to him. He said let me show you where this fragrant odor is coming from! He showed me a steel pit on the floor and around this circular pit was a protective rim about one foot high. This was the largest and loudest garbage disposal I had ever seen! Everything in the pit was red and there was a terrible grinding gurgling sound, sucking everything down into the red ooze! Just then, a large panel truck backed in. All the workers guided the truck into position. When the truck door flung open a great mass of flies took to the air. It looked like a black swarm of bees. They landed everywhere. The workers and I were covered with flies! The Chief was watching my reaction to all that was happening. Then, the workers pickup long polls with sharp hooks on the end. They began pulling off dead bodies of animals and let them drop into the swirling red ooze in the disposal! What a sound of grinding and gurgling I heard! As I looked up to see, what was going to happen next, I noticed everyone was looking at me. They continue pulling all of the animals off the truck and it pulled out. The mass of grinding ooze was now covered with about eight inches of blood. I thought it would overflow the steel barrier. One of the workers nudged me and joking saying, "Don't slip and fall in there now!

The boss waved his hand and said let me show you where you're going to work. I thought at least that it's not in the disposal room. I walked along behind him as he pointed out different noteworthy locations. Everything just smelled something awful! The chief said I would actually get use to the smell. I surely didn't know when that would happen. Finally, we entered a very large room painted a light green. There were boxes of dog food stacked literally to the ceiling. All I could see was row after row and stack after stack. I thought I'd be loading these boxes into a truck with a forklift. Not even a close guess! The boss started down on a small stack of boxes. He said, "Do you see that mess?" I said, "Yes." He said, "It happens all the time. The cans just don't seem to get filled right and first thing, you know 'BANG,' one of the cans exploded all over the place. The explosions are so strong they rip those shipping boxes all apart." I was thinking to myself that I brought a lunch. He told me to put my lunch box in one of those lockers. He said, now what you are going to be doing, is inspecting each case of dog food in this room. The good ones just send them back on the conveyer belt. The cases with problems; you take all of the bad cans out of the boxes and put them on this conveyer belt. All the cans that are still acceptable take them out of the box and send them back on this conveyer belt. Now the last thing is, on that far wall is the conveyer belt, where bad cases will be coming in for you to work on. I told him that I understood and would do my best.

What kind of mess did I get myself into this time? I worked until afternoon break and everyone was heading to the back loading dock so, I tagged along. We made pleasant conversation; they asked me all kinds of questions about, where I was from and things that I had done.

As we were talking, I opened my lunch box and much to my surprise, my sandwiches were black! I couldn't believe my eyes. I had no idea what the problem could be. I pulled out a sandwich and started to remove it from the baggy. It was covered in little bugs! I showed it to the man next to me and he laughed as he said, "Those are just fleas, they don't eat much!" I threw my whole lunch box into the trashcan. He said, "Now, you can see why most of us just go to the tavern across the street and drink our lunch."

Well, it was about closing time, so I headed over to the office looking for the boss. I walked into his office and what I was feeling must have been written all over my face. I told the Chief about what I thought and told him that he could keep my paycheck for the day, because this had been a real education. I thanked him for his understanding, and I left. The Chief was laughing saying; "I told you this wasn't the job for you!"

When I got home to my relatives house, I told them of my experience. They thought it was a good idea not to take the job. I waited until my two-week stay was over and I told them I would have to go, I've stayed long enough. I thanked them for their assistance and ideas about jobs. I told them I would head back to Maryland and look for a job there.

I didn't plan to stay at my birth mothers house and I didn't have an apartment pick out yet. I had a few things on my mind about my own ability to make ends meet. I was use to traveling out of a sea bag, so this didn't seem so bad.

As I returned from the trip to my relative's house, I thought it might be nice to stop in and see how one of my siblings was doing. She was married, had two kids, and lived in a big high-rise apartment complex. Things looked ok from the outside, but I wouldn't find out until much later, that there was trouble in paradise. She said nothing to me about any type of problems she had, but she told me that my younger brother was living in his car down in the underground parking garage. I was very surprised and concerned.

I went down to find him; I was looking for a white valiant. I found him on the last level down over in a far corner of the underground parking lot. I talked to him for a while and found out he has been living in his car for about six months. I made a deal with him that if he got a job, he and I could move in to an apartment together. I made sure he understood he would have to pay his half. He thought that was great.

I recently received the results back from the Civil Service and I passed the test. I was rated as a GS-4. I went to the Naval Communications Station and got a job that day. Things looked like they were going to work out. My younger brother and I picked out an apartment together. He got a job as a kitchen helper at a fancy restaurant. From 1968 to 1972, I drank I guess, because that's what everyone in the military did to relax. This habit continued over into my civilian life. The property owner of the apartment complex said we were the nosiest and most problematic tenements she ever had! This nice woman liked us for some reason; I really do not know why? She didn't kick us out for making too much noise.

My younger brother met a girl and she moved in with him. I was seeing a cute girl, but I wouldn't let her move in with me until we were married. I guess I'm old fashion. In 1973, June 29, my wife and I got married and by some miracle, we have stayed together until the present. Now, my younger brother, that I helped find a place to live, skipped out on the rent, moved to Delaware, and got married on the very same day that we did. We have always thought that to be strange. We preformed many good deeds for people in need. Then they would shaft us afterwards. This has always been a mystery to us! We have never stopped giving assistance to those that need it.

Oh! Bye the way, the resident manager woman that liked us, came to speak to my wife and told her she was so thankful the boys were married and settled down a lot.

From 1973 to 1977, my wife and I lived in apartments in Maryland. From 1973 to 1977, drinking became a way of live. Anyone that knows me very well, I'm the kind of person that takes everything to its maximum limit. Well that's the same way I was when I was drinking. This was something that had to change or it would wreck by marriage.

My very youngest brother was living with us for a year. He spent his entire time partying, drinking, and smoking weed. I gave him four choices: Go to school, Go to work, Go in the Military Service, or get out. He made his decision that week and entered the U.S. Navy. The next time we heard about him was from a knock on the door. It was the Shore Patrol from U.S. Navy; they were looking for my A.W.O.L. youngest brother. We told them we hadn't heard from him. We would call if we see him.

When we got the news that we were having a baby in 1976, I knew the drinking had to change. That knowledge came with much long-suffering and prompting from my wife. I thought to help me change things; I would enroll in computer school at night. Our daughter was born in September, and I graduated from school in March of 1977.

I got a job in Virginia and I decided, without very much consultation with my wife we moved to an apartment in Virginia. It was located halfway between both of our jobs. From 1977 to 1980, we lived in a Virginia apartment. I was cutting out all visits to my family members, because they all drank heavily. I was trying to get my life headed in a new direction. I had a new career, apartment, and a new beginning. Well, by the beginning of 1978, I had given up drinking. Now, I picked up a new habit to replace it.

From 1978 to 1980, I join an occult church. As always, I took it to the limit. I read almost every book they printed, the Bible, and even a few more. I studied under a Minister with PHD. I was completely immersed in this new way of thinking and how to act as a responsible adult. In 1980, my wife and I separated and she moved in with her mom at the farmhouse. It was a beautiful setting, away from the activity of the city, but local enough to commute to work each day.

I didn't know what to think or what to do about my situation. I had cut off all ties to all of my family members. I had no one to turn to except the members of the church. For two months, I prayed and thought over the beliefs, I held. I thought about the path of life I was taking. Then, this little old woman came to talk to me one day. She said something very simple and then went away. She said, "Remember, anything that separates a husband from a wife is not correct!" I saw her at church a few times after that; she never said another word. She had that look of remember what I said. After two months, I had enough of the advisement from all the people in the church that I could handle.

Now, for these two months I had not called by wife, because I didn't know what to say. I had no proposal of how to fix this problem. I prayed all I could pray, but the only thing that stuck in my head was the words from the old woman. I had such a heavy weight pressing down upon me to take some action. I finally called my wife and asked for visitation with my daughter. My wife agreed and I began to see my daughter on the weekends.

The pressure on me would not relent. I felt compelled to take the next big step to turn my life around. I updated my resume and sent it to companies in Maryland. I immediately received a response for an interview. I got the job. I packed up everything that I had and moved to a location that I knew would be expectable to my wife.

We were separated for eleven month. I had asked her for nine months what did she need for be to do. What changes could we make? I told her I left the church months ago. I told her I was working and living in Maryland. What else could I do? I asked her many times to reconcile, but she said she was not comfortable with me and still afraid. I was at the end of my rope. I didn't have a clue about how to change this situation. I was out of answers. At this point, I began to give up.

The last three months, I was so despondent; I was in a living hell! I didn't like feeling this way and I really didn't have to live like this if I didn't want to. I began making detailed plans to kill myself. With my personality, there was no doing it halfway; it would be all or nothing. I had decided that I could not take the pain, pressure, and feeling the way I did anymore! I had planned everything out, the date, and the location. All I need now was the gun! I was sitting in my apartment and I was getting ready to go get the gun. After spending two years in a war, I knew what the feeling of death was. I was standing right at the edge of the door.

When, the phone rang, it was my wife said she would like to meet with me. Of course, I said yes. Even today, I don't know how things came out right. I'm definitely sure it wasn't my ideas, because I didn't have an answer to spare. When people ask me how it feels to stand at the edge of the brink of death, I just tell them you don't want to feel it or even be there! Along with our reunion, we decided that we would all go to family counseling. We wanted to find out what was wrong and do our best to make it right!

We started our new life in a town house apartment. This wasn't a problem; we just wanted our own home. For our reunion my wife, daughter, and I drove to Disney World in Florida and stayed for a couple of days. That was a time to remember.

Then it was 1982, the year we had been waiting for a long time. We bought our first house. It was a handy-man special. It was ours. I was the handy man. The first time we came to the house we were going to clean it up. Boy, did we have a job. I'm wandering if I should tell the whole story. I'll try it; I can always delete it, right. Oh! Well! Here it goes.

On a sunny day in June, we proudly opened the door to our wonderful new thirty-year-old house. We came to clean, but looking at each other, we asked where that smell is coming from. With a quick check of the house, we knew where the smell was not. We returned to the living room and we knew something was definitely here. We checked the wall-to-wall carpeting and it was damp. We looked about for any obvious water leaks and we found none. My wife said the rug smells! The whole crew lifted and folded back the rug. We looked at each other and said there is another rug. The top rug really smelled, so we pulled it up and dumped it in the front yard. Now, the second rug was damp, so we lifted it up and pitched it in the front yard. Then, we found that a third rug was also damp. We pulled that rug up and my eye really opened wide! There had to be at least a billion bugs and that's no lie. We throw the third rug out. Then, we began using a dustpan and broom to crape up all of the live bugs running everywhere. We got all that we could catch and filled half of a Pepsi box of bugs. They went out front. There was still a smelly liquid floating on the floor. After talking to the neighbors, we found out it was dog urine. Boy, were we having fun now! Now we understood what it meant to be a "Happy Home Owner." I'll tell you it was not funny!

We didn't sleep in the house until all the bugs were dead. Each day I set off bug bombs in every room on every floor. Then we had Terminex come in and fumigate the insides of the walls. The next three days that house saw more than it share of bug bombs, Pinesol, Mr. Clean, Lestoil, and lots of cleaning fluids. I sure was glad that we had a strong health crew to help us get past the grime and down to the shine.

Once we got the cleaning and other details finished, it was time to paint. We decided to paint everything, ceiling to floor. We threw it out, we dumped it out, we scrubbed it out, and we bomb it out, so now it was time seal it out. This was our first house and my wife and I decided on a set of colors that we like to use in each room. To help everyone out we put the correct paint color in each room. All the supplies they would need. Everything was going alone perfectly until my wife told me my birth mother was painting our daughter's room the color she wanted. I went to check and wouldn't you know it, she took the paint from another room. It was my mother so it was my place to talk to her and explain what was wrong.

Well, I walked in and said just checking things out. How are you doing in here? Do you have everything you need? She said yes and she was doing fine. I looked at what she was painting and politically correct, I told her that I must have given her the wrong color of paint. Wait and I'll get you the correct color. That's when she said; I'm going to paint it my color. Slowly I was building up steam. Mother, I said, Margie wants the room painted blue! Mother, I said the room is going to be blue! My mother said, don't use that tone with me! I looked her right in the eye and said, don't you understand that this is Margie's house and she has already chosen what the colors will be! My mother said she'd paint it whatever color she wanted to! By this time, my patients were gone and my volume was turned on high. Four-letter words that I forgot I knew started flying out of my mouth. I didn't even give her time to speak. I told her what I thought about her paint job, her personality, her team spirit, and a bunch more things. I told her to get her aaaas out of this house and don't come back. She flew out the front door and got in her car, slammed the car door and took off down the road at top speed. You know she never did come back. My wife and I didn't mind at all!

Everyone was frozen in his or her assigned rooms. The loud conflict echoed through the empty house! We were yelling so load that I didn't have to explain anything. I could feel the tension in the air. All of the people there knew my birth mother. For her to go off was nothing new. I turned up the music in the living room and everyone settled back to his or her jobs.

As we settled in, I made taking care of the home my hobby. About a week after we bought the house, a terrible storm came, tore down our shed, blew the basement window in, and it fell on the furnace oil line and drained 150 gallon of fuel oil into the basement. We used a lot of kitty litter to soak up the oil and you know that really works. Months later, the lightning hit a tree in the back and it fell on the house. The lightning also hit the air conditioner compressor out side and burned it up. I could see this hobby of taking care of the house could become very complicated and expensive.

My wife says I was very neat and particular about everything. She says I was a perfectionist. For the first three years, there was just so much to do, that I really stayed busy. I had a lot of energy back in those days. For two years, I cut down thirteen, thirty-foot pine trees. I cut up the trunks and used them for six years of firewood. That saved us a bunch of money. I painted the house every year.

We had many picnics for all the kids. As you know when you have kids, you have the neighbor kids too. We had a very nice time. It never was a burden to host the other children. Our basement was a completely open space, with a concrete floor. It was a very nice play area, once all the oil was cleaned up. All of my daughter's friends would come over to roller skate in the basement. They would have a great time swinging around on the metal pillars that held up the house. It was a nice cool place for the kids to play and we always knew where they were.

We also, setup swings and a slide in the shaded part of the yard. After taking out the trees and replacing the surface with grass, the children had almost an acre of fenced area where they could safely play. We also, had two eighty-pound Alaskan huskies to keep the children company.

We planted new trees and built our own brick patio. We built a wooden fence around the front, planted flowers, and put in flowerbeds. Don't get me wrong, all of these things transpired over twelve to fifteen years. This didn't happen all at once.

I would help with the laundry, wash, and polish the vehicles. My hobby was remodeling the complete basement. I wanted to do all the work myself.

In 1988, we purchased a runabout boat. For three years, we took to boat out with the children to fish and just ride the river. When I say the kids, I mean my daughter, our niece and three nephews. We had helped, supported, and raised them since 1974. We just thought of them as part of the family.

Each summer we tried to provide some type of activity that would make the summer a memorable time for the kids. One year I drove my daughter and my wife from Maryland to Minnesota. The non-stop trip took a little over thirty hours. We had an exciting time in the land of 10,000 lakes. Another summer trip my wife, my daughter, the three cousins, and I went on a trip where we visited all of the caves in Virginia. That trip was even educational for me. A few times my wife and I drove the kids from Maryland to Indiana, where their Aunt and Uncle picked them up for the other half of the trip to Minnesota. They had a splendid summer vacation there.

We Took In Friends and Relatives Down On Their Luck

Since my wife and I have been married, we have always helped those in need. We believe if there is a person down on their luck and we have the means to help them, then we helped. It could be a need of food, cloths, and shelter, no matter what we believed it was our duty to help. Of course we didn't do this blindly, we expected the person in need to do their part. Let me tell you about a few events and then I'll tell you what happened.

We loaned money to my wife's sister, so she could get a truck to transport the children. Well, she never paid the money back, we cosigned for the loan, and the truck was repossessed.

One of my brothers wife died, he was an alcoholic, had to go to treatment, he lost his job because of the drinking, had no car, and had to sell his house. Now I would say this person is down on their luck. We let him move in with us.

He lived with us for two years. We were his scoffer until he got a car. After a few months in recovery, he got a job. He never bought food or paid any rent. We were patient with him as long as we could. Then, when we told him what his rent would be each month, he immediately moved out. He had saved enough money to put a large down payment on a new house. We sold him our car hoping that would help him out. Unbelievably, within a month he sold the car for twice the amount we sold it to him. I guess we should have sold it to him for full price. I don't think I'll ever understand people.

We were struggling to make ends meet. We learned a few things from that experience. Oh! Bye the way, we haven't seen or heard from him since. That must be ten or so years ago. This is very puzzling to us!

My half-sister was having problems at home during her teenage years. I talked with my mother and told her that maybe things would go better, if she got a little space for a while. She stayed with us for six months of hell. She had so many problems even I don't know where to start. After six months, we sent her back home. A wise person knows when to step back.

We had a father and mother with a child down on their luck. They need a place to live and save money to get back on their feet. This experience lasted one year and I had to make them leave. The first incident was the father smacking the child with all his strength. I immediately called him on it and told him child abuse of any kind would not be tolerated. I told him if it happens again pack your bags. The second and final incident happened when all the children were playing in the back yard. The father tied a toy car with a six-foot rope to a dog. It was very frightening to watch the dog fly around the yard very fast, with the toy car and child tumbling behind it. That was it! After the child was safe, I told them to move out immediately.

His mother threw one of our nephews out of the house and we took the teenage boy into our house. He was a good kid trying to go the right way. We enrolled him in the same church school where we sent our daughter. He seemed to be doing well. After nine months, he told us he wanted to leave and return home. The reason he was going home is his mother told him she was sorry for throwing him out and that she should have known better. She is an alcoholic. He was torn between the truth and the reality of the situation he would face at home. We told him he was free to make his own choice. He went back home. He has expressed regret, to us, about his decision.

We currently have our brother-in-law living with us. He's working very hard to get his life together. He and my half-sister are divorced. Well, we have heard through the grapevine that the whole family was avoiding us, because we allow him to live with us. I told him years before if he ever needed help, call us and we would see what we could do. He has lived with us for three years and we have had no problems with him.

We know better. The whole family has avoided us for all kinds of other reasons for over twenty-eight years. The word I'm looking for is; they are all superficial friends. Another thing that is funny, we haven't heard from many of our friends since I became ill with PTSD. My wife and I have learned many valuable lessons.

How Is Work Before And After PTSD?

Now, the last item I want to discuss is work before PTSD. I was a Computer Scientist. My work was always demanding and very stressful. This is really no surprise to me. I know when you have a job where many personnel are depending on the completion of a decision you have to make, is a stressful job.

From 1990-1995, the level of stress for me went off the charts. My belief was that I was handling the stress ok. My mind, body, and nervous system told me otherwise. When the stress seemed stronger, I pushed a little harder giving it my all. My mind, body, and nervous system completely shutdown automatically on

May 10, 1995. Complete control has not returned for my use yet, but I'm moving forward.

How is work after PTSD? I'm categorized as completely disabled. PTSD is an extraordinary illness to deal with. I have both physical and mental symptoms or impairments that appear and disappear automatically. Mentally I cannot force these symptoms to cease. Writing, positive thinking or medications haven't returned the control of my mind and body to me. PTSD is at the time of this writing an incurable disorder. The best I can hope for is to use coping skills to bring peace, safety, and sanity to my life's endeavors.

Not all is glum and doom! It's a delight finding that coping skills are the most dependable medium to continue my gradually recovery! Controlling my reaction to the symptoms has shown positive results! Keep working on coping skills.

Presently I have not attained my highest goal of holding down a nine to five job. With a positive attitude, I'm always working toward some type of part time employment to sustain my family and so should you. Good luck on your journey, don't give up!

About The Author

Phil Dorman one of four boys in a family of five children, endured nine years of extreme brutality at the hands of his parents. Even in the midst of such sadistic abuse, he took on the responsibility of parenting, feeding, and protecting the children the best a nine-year-old boy could. He persevered, driven only by his loyalty to the children, until he left home at eighteen years of age.

He served four honorable years, as a radioman in the U.S. Navy. He is a Decorated Vietnam Veteran of two years of combat duty. His patriotism continued after the war, he continued his education, while working for the Department of Defense on Telecommunications projects for five years. Over the next twenty years, he continued attending school at night. As a Computer Scientist, he worked on critical projects for the Department of the Navy. He received many letters of commendation for his work related to Desert Storm, Desert Shield, and the U.S. efforts in the Somalian Crisis.

He is fifty-four years old, has an extremely long-suffering wife, one beautiful daughter, a great son-in-law, and one wonderful grandson.

Phil Dorman acquired firsthand knowledge about all types of work related stress, physical and mental abuse, and combat trauma. He endured nine years of child abuse and trauma, he served bravely two years of combat trauma, and he spent twenty-nine years working on extremely time critical stressful projects as a Computer Scientist for the Department Of Defense.

After forty years of abuse, trauma, extreme stress he became ill with acute Post Traumatic Stress Disorder (PTSD), May 10, 1995. Struggling for nine years, he's arrived at a stage of gradual recovery. It wasn't until December of 2001, that he was able to begin writing his incredible story. Though he still suffers from acute PTSD, he has utilized every available resource to make this book available to all of the people suffering from child abuse, trauma, Veterans of combat trauma, and PTSD.

His hope is that, "I Cry For Help!" will reduce the fear and suffering of others through the real-life experiences contained in this book.

Book Summary

My name is Phil Dorman and I would like to share some knowledge with you. I have Post Traumatic Stress Disorder (PTSD) and Dissociative Disorders (DD). These disorders caused through sadistic child abuse, childhood trauma, normal stress, trauma due to combat actions, and overworking for thirty years, have plagued me for over nine years. Not a doctor or in the medical professional, you might say I'm writing from on the inside. Without a formal degree in pain, trauma, stress, and suffering, unless the count of forty years of actual personal experience is considered, I too am searching for answers. Many have learned through actual experiences and spending six years of my life almost totally locked up in my mind, may just qualify as unsurpassed wisdom. With my vow to increase the knowledge base for the common person about PTSD and its causes, patiently I waited for my reprieve from this dungeon. Thinking that this information would help to bring order and logic for loved ones to see, understand, and begin to cope with some of the problems that can devastate a family from these disorders. Coping, the most powerful process, the whole family can learn about any disease or a disorder brings a sense of calm during a mighty storm. These disorders have torn both my immediate and extended family apart. This knowledge can produce a more favorable outcome for your family. You need knowledge in order to take action.

When suffering at my lowest point, there was nothing to read in simple English to help me through this overwhelming trauma called PTSD. Any family doesn't have the ability to help their loved one cope or understand without the proper knowledge. The person with PTSD can't always understand or cope with current events. The person that has undergone this rapid neurological change is mentally fragile and unstable at best. The person can comprehend small bits and pieces of information. The person may appear to have a foreign persona to all that knew them. In the beginning, the person requires time to absorb the physical changes to them. Panic and terror permeates every cell of their body! Scared to death is a mild way of saying how my beginning felt! Terrified by questions and answers was the only activity on my mind. Some of my questions were; what was the cause of my illness? What was happening to me? How do I correct this problem? Am I going to die? Am I going crazy? Where shall I begin? Will I be like this forever? My mind was continually flooded with racing thoughts.

Of course, the severity of PTSD is different for each person. I've been in combat and PTSD was more terrifying to me than a sneak attack. No abilities did I posses to understand the simple things of life happening around me. Some examples are; people talking, hearing sounds, all of the senses, and physical motor skills. My view was from the dungeon in my mind.

"I Cry For Help," but no one hears me. No one could read what I wrote. I was about to explode; what was I going to do? Whom could I trust? Everything felt so strange in my paranoid state. Could I trust my wife? Was she was going to poison me? Would the men in the white coats take me away! In this book, I give real life illustrations of the symptoms associated with PTSD. Moreover, these examples can help the families to understand and cope with everyday situations. In September 2003, my diagnosis of Bipolar Disorder requires additional coping skills. My completed research on this subject will become available shortly.

A Tribute To My Best Friend

I would like to give thanks to a very special friend. She stayed with me everyday and night, during this long illness. She died on October 3, 2001. She taught me about love and devotion. She was selfless, as no other one I've known. She would guard me always, no one got past her weary eyes. She would always be by my side and kept me warm on many a wintry night. She would not even go to eat or go out to the bathroom, until her sister came to relieve her from guard duty, across the bedroom doorway. When my watch rang out signaling it was time to take my medicine. She would bite the side of my watch to turn off the alarm. Then, she would gently lick my eyelids, to wake me up to take my next prescription pill. She even took me on my daily, one mile, walks. Even when it was summer and quite hot outside, we enjoyed just walking slowly, but there was still that burst of excitement each time she saw a squirrel. I remember how beautifully she howled to her favorite country song. She kept me going, when nothing else would. I've thought about her often over the months she's been gone. I had her with me a little over ten years. My best friend was ALASKA. I've always thought that her name showed that she could brave the elements and still keep going strong. Alaska was a gentle female; weighing eighty pounds, before she got ill. She was sick for about a year and I stayed by her side, through it all. I have a little feeling inside that believes she gave me her energy, just before she left. Alaska was a very special person to me. I feel she had a spirit and personality all her own. She never was, just an animal to me. She was a person that cared for me. She gave me an abundance of love and affection, over her ten years. She was red, white, and stood proudly waist high. She was my great big Honey Bear. She always had a smile and she talked with a soft growl to me. She never was cross with me and she was surprisingly gentle for a large Siberian husky. Alaska, I'll always love you and will never forget you for the rest of my life. Good Bye My Friend, You Truly Were My Honey Bears!
My Best Friend

Acknowledgments

Thanks to God for control over my disorders, guidance, and inspiration to write this book.

Thanks to Grandma W. for all those home cooked meal with wonderful butter biscuits.

To my loving Soul Mate of thirty-two years my solace that guide me during desperate times! I want to thank my wife for unwavering support, understanding, and delight all my life.

To Dr. Ralph W. Wadeson, Jr., M.D. Psychiatry, I salute publicly for his undying support and dedication that brought me to this level of gradual recovery. Without doctors of his caliber the community would truly suffer a greatly lose. He has utilized the current technology to its fullest and restored me to a whole human being. I tip my hat to you sir! Receiving control of my mind again, is a wonderful gift, which I will treasure for the rest of my life!

To our dearest friend D.R. we give enormous thanks for showing us the deep meanings of being a true Good Samaritan. She seemed to know where our lives would turn next and with long-sufferingly she awaited for our arrival. We often call her our Guardian Angel, for in our heart she truly has earned the name through love. She's supplied our need more than we can express or ever repay.

To my loving daughter (my Midget), grandson, and son-in-law for tolerant listening, telling jokes to make me laugh. We thank them all for their endless editing, household chores, construction, shoveling two feet of snow from the roof, courage, love, and lasting family support.

To my grandson I offer special thanks for helping me endure the experience at The Wall. He shows me every day how to use and repair the child within me. This special little guy has helped me find funny stories in my past. We thank them both for taking the time to teach our grandson how to be a child. He will see the world as it should be!

We give thanks to our brother-in-law for his continual support and belief in our ability to snap back from this devastation.

Endorsement

Endorsement From: Ralph W. Wadeson, Jr., M.D. Psychiatry

I am Ralph W. Wadeson, Jr., M.D. Psychiatry. Attended Emory University and the Medical College of Alabama, I received my MD in 1947. Working as a County Doctor in Alabama from 1948 to 1952, my service to my country began as a Battalion Surgeon with the US Marine Corp in Korea from 1952 to 1954. In 1954, I joined the Psychiatry Department of Hines V.A. Hospital, transferred to the Psychiatry Department of Michael Reese Hospital of Chicago in 1955, and stayed until 1958. Continuing I work in research for the National Institute Mental Health from 1958 to 1960.

Phil Dorman and I have worked together for nine long arduous years. My opinion that Phil Dorman has both the knowledge and experience required to present the information in this book. These true stories tell of extremely traumatic events from a patient with Post Traumatic Stress Disorder (PTSD). There is no other book in print today; that contains the details of such events, with strong, sensitive, and graphic language. This book details the failures, struggles, attempts, and successes that Phil Dorman has documented in his written journals for nine years.

I have read this book and recommend it as valuable reading to the families dealing with trauma, child abuse trauma, combat trauma, extreme stress, or PTSD.

I would like to join Phil Dorman in the hope that this book, "I Cry For Help!" will relieve some of the pain and suffering caused by different traumatic disorders.

The End—Of "*I Cry For Help!*"

978-0-595-40961-7
0-595-40961-X

www.ingramcontent.com/pod-product-compliance
Lightning Source LLC
Chambersburg PA
CBHW020436290526
45785CB00002B/871